ABC OF
LIVER, PANCREAS AND GALL BLADDER

ABC OF LIVER, PANCREAS AND GALL BLADDER

Edited by

I J BECKINGHAM

Consultant Hepatobiliary and Laparoscopic Surgeon, Queen's Medical Centre, Nottingham

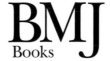

© BMJ Books 2001
BMJ Books is an imprint of the BMJ Publishing Group

First published in 2001
by BMJ Books, BMA House, Tavistock Square,
London WC1H 9JR

www.bmjbooks.com

British Library Cataloguing in Publication Data

A catalogue record for this book is available from the British Library

ISBN 0 7279 1531 2

Cover design by Marritt Associates, Harrow, Middlesex
Typeset by FiSH Books and BMJ Electronic Production

Printed and bound in Spain by GraphyCems, Navarra

Contents

Contributors

I J Beckingham
Consultant Hepatobiliary and Laparoscopic Surgeon,
Queen's Medical Centre, Nottingham

P C Bornman
Professor of Surgery, University of Cape Town, South
Africa

J E J Krige
Associate Professor of Surgery, Groote Schuur
Hospital, Cape Town, South Africa

J P A Lodge
Consultant Hepatobiliary and Transplant Surgeon, St
James Hospital, Leeds

K R Prasad
Senior Transplant Fellow, St James Hospital, Leeds

S D Ryder
Consultant Hepatologist, Queen's Medical Centre,
Nottingham

Preface

Diseases of the Liver, Pancreas and biliary system affect a substantial proportion of the worlds population and involve doctors and health care workers across many disciplines. Many of these diseases produce great misery and distress and are economically important requiring much time off work. The aim of this series was to provide an overview of these diseases and enable the busy clinician to keep abreast of advances in diagnosis and management of not only the common but also the rarer, but none the less important, conditions.

1 Investigation of liver and biliary disease

I J Beckingham, S D Ryder

Jaundice is the commonest presentation of patients with liver and biliary disease. The cause can be established in most cases by simple non-invasive tests, but many patients will require referral to a specialist for management. Patients with high concentrations of bilirubin (>100 μmol/l) or with evidence of sepsis or cholangitis are at high risk of developing complications and should be referred as an emergency because delays in treatment adversely affect prognosis.

Jaundice

Hyperbilirubinaemia is defined as a bilirubin concentration above the normal laboratory upper limit of 19 μmol/l. Jaundice occurs when bilirubin becomes visible within the sclera, skin, and mucous membranes, at a blood concentration of around 40 μmol/l. Jaundice can be categorised as prehepatic, hepatic, or posthepatic, and this provides a useful framework for identifying the underlying cause.

Around 3% of the UK population have hyperbilirubinaemia (up to 100 μmol/l) caused by excess unconjugated bilirubin, a condition known as Gilbert's syndrome. These patients have mild impairment of conjugation within the hepatocytes. The condition usually becomes apparent only during a transient rise in bilirubin concentration (precipitated by fasting or illness) that results in frank jaundice. Investigations show an isolated unconjugated hyperbilirubinaemia with normal liver enzyme activities and reticulocyte concentrations. The syndrome is often familial and does not require treatment.

Prehepatic jaundice
In prehepatic jaundice, excess unconjugated bilirubin is produced faster than the liver is able to conjugate it for excretion. The liver can excrete six times the normal daily load before bilirubin concentrations in the plasma rise. Unconjugated bilirubin is insoluble and is not excreted in the urine. It is most commonly due to increased haemolysis—for example, in spherocytosis, homozygous sickle cell disease, or thalassaemia major—and patients are often anaemic with splenomegaly. The cause can usually be determined by further haematological tests (red cell film for reticulocytes and abnormal red cell shapes, haemoglobin electrophoresis, red cell antibodies, and osmotic fragility).

Hepatic and posthepatic jaundice
Most patients with jaundice have hepatic (parenchymal) or posthepatic (obstructive) jaundice. Several clinical features may help distinguish these two important groups but cannot be relied on, and patients should have ultrasonography to look for evidence of biliary obstruction.

The most common intrahepatic causes are viral hepatitis, alcoholic cirrhosis, primary biliary cirrhosis, drug induced jaundice, and alcoholic hepatitis. Posthepatic jaundice is most often due to biliary obstruction by a stone in the common bile duct or by carcinoma of the pancreas. Pancreatic pseudocyst, chronic pancreatitis, sclerosing cholangitis, a bile duct stricture, or parasites in the bile duct are less common causes.

In obstructive jaundice (both intrahepatic cholestasis and extrahepatic obstruction) the serum bilirubin is principally conjugated. Conjugated bilirubin is water soluble and is

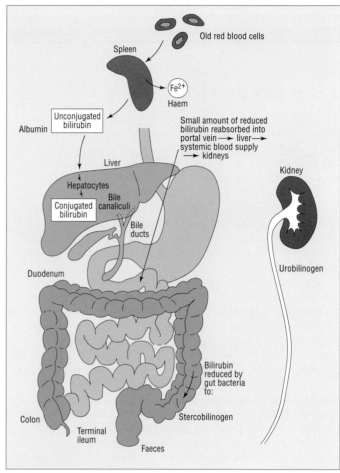

Figure 1.1 Bilirubin pathway

Box 1.1 History that should be taken from patients presenting with jaundice
- Duration of jaundice
- Previous attacks of jaundice
- Pain
- Chills, fever, systemic symptoms
- Itching
- Exposure to drugs (prescribed and illegal)
- Biliary surgery
- Anorexia, weight loss
- Colour of urine and stool
- Contact with other jaundiced patients
- History of injections or blood transfusions
- Occupation

Box1.2 Examination of patients with jaundice
- Depth of jaundice
- Scratch marks
- Signs of chronic liver disease:
  Palmar erythema
  Clubbing
  White nails
  Dupuytren's contracture
  Gynaecomastia
- Liver:
  Size
  Shape
  Surface
- Enlargement of gall bladder
- Splenomegaly
- Abdominal mass
- Colour of urine and stools

excreted in the urine, giving it a dark colour (bilirubinuria). At the same time, lack of bilirubin entering the gut results in pale, "putty" coloured stools and an absence of urobilinogen in the urine when measured by dipstick testing. Jaundice due to hepatic parenchymal disease is characterised by raised concentrations of both conjugated and unconjugated serum bilirubin, and typically stools and urine are of normal colour. However, although pale stools and dark urine are a feature of biliary obstruction, they can occur transiently in many acute hepatic illnesses and are therefore not a reliable clinical feature to distinguish obstruction from hepatic causes of jaundice.

Liver function tests

Liver function tests routinely combine markers of function (albumin and bilirubin) with markers of liver damage (alanine transaminase, alkaline phosphatase, and γ-glutamyl transferase). Abnormalities in liver enzyme activities give useful information about the nature of the liver insult: a predominant rise in alanine transaminase activity (normally contained within the hepatocytes) suggests a hepatic process. Serum transaminase activity is not usually raised in patients with obstructive jaundice, although in patients with common duct stones and cholangitis a mixed picture of raised biliary and hepatic enzyme activity is often seen.

Epithelial cells lining the bile canaliculi produce alkaline phosphatase, and its serum activity is raised in patients with intrahepatic cholestasis, cholangitis, or extrahepatic obstruction; increased activity may also occur in patients with focal hepatic lesions in the absence of jaundice. In cholangitis with incomplete extrahepatic obstruction, patients may have normal or slightly raised serum bilirubin concentrations and high serum alkaline phosphatase activity. Serum alkaline phosphatase is also produced in bone, and bone disease may complicate the interpretation of abnormal alkaline phosphatase activity. If increased activity is suspected to be from bone, serum concentrations of calcium and phosphorus should be measured together with 5′-nucleotidase or γ-glutamyl transferase activity; these two enzymes are also produced by bile ducts, and their activity is raised in cholestasis but remains unchanged in bone disease.

Occasionally, the enzyme abnormalities may not give a clear answer, showing both a biliary and hepatic component. This is usually because of cholangitis associated with stones in the common bile duct, where obstruction is accompanied by hepatocyte damage as a result of infection within the biliary tree.

Plasma proteins and coagulation factors

A low serum albumin concentration suggests chronic liver disease. Most patients with biliary obstruction or acute hepatitis will have normal serum albumin concentrations as the half life of albumin in plasma is around 20 days and it takes at least 10 days for the concentration to fall below the normal range despite impaired liver function.

Coagulation factors II, V, VII, and IX are synthesised in the liver. Abnormal clotting (measured as prolongation of the international normalised ratio) occurs in both biliary obstruction and parenchymal liver disease because of a combination of poor absorption of fat soluble vitamin K (due to absence of bile in the gut) and a reduced ability of damaged hepatocytes to produce clotting factors.

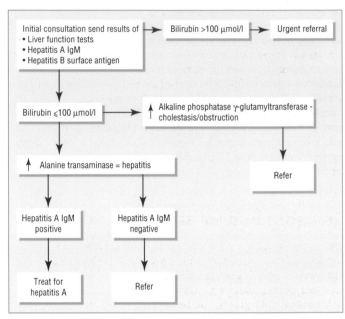

Figure 1.2 Guide to investigation and referral of patients with jaundice in primary care

Box 1.3 Drugs that may cause liver damage

Analgesics
- Paracetamol
- Aspirin
- Non-steroidal anti-inflammatory drugs

Cardiac drugs
- Methyldopa
- Amiodarone

Psychotropic drugs
- Monoamine oxidase inhibitors
- Phenothiazines (such as chlorpromazine)

Others
- Sodium valproate
- Oestrogens (oral contraceptives and hormone replacement therapy)

The presence of a low serum albumin concentration in a jaundiced patient suggests a chronic disease process

Serum globulin titres rise in chronic hepatitis and cirrhosis, mainly due to a rise in the IgA and IgG fractions. High titres of IgM are characteristic of primary biliary cirrhosis, and IgG is a hallmark of chronic active hepatitis. Ceruloplasmin activity (ferroxidase, a copper transporting globulin) is reduced in Wilson's disease. Deficiency of α_1 antitrypsin (an enzyme inhibitor) is a cause of cirrhosis as well as emphysema. High concentrations of the iron carrying protein ferritin are a marker of haemochromatosis.

Autoantibodies are a series of antibodies directed against subcellular fractions of various organs that are released into the circulation when cells are damaged. High titres of antimitochondrial antibodies are specific for primary biliary cirrhosis, and antismooth muscle and antinuclear antibodies are often seen in autoimmune chronic active hepatitis. Antibodies against hepatitis are discussed in detail in a future article on hepatitis.

Table 1.1 Autoantibody and immunoglobulin characteristics in liver disease

	Autoantibodies	Immunoglobulins
Primary biliary cirrhosis	High titre of antimitochondrial antibody in 95% of patients	Raised IgM
Autoimmune chronic active hepatitis	Smooth muscle antibody in 70%, antinuclear factor in 60%, Low antimitochondrial antibody titre in 20%	Raised IgG in all patients
Primary sclerosing cholangitis	Antinuclear cytoplasmic antibody in 30%	

Imaging in liver and biliary disease

Plain radiography has a limited role in the investigation of hepatobiliary disease. Chest radiography may show small amounts of subphrenic gas, abnormalities of diaphragmatic contour, and related pulmonary disease, including metastases. Abdominal radiographs can be useful if a patient has calcified or gas containing lesions as these may be overlooked or misinterpreted on ultrasonography. Such lesions include calcified gall stones (10-15% of gall stones), chronic calcific pancreatitis, gas containing liver abscesses, portal venous gas, and emphysematous cholecystitis.

Ultrasonography is the first line imaging investigation in patients with jaundice, right upper quadrant pain, or hepatomegaly. It is non-invasive, inexpensive, and quick but requires experience in technique and interpretation. Ultrasonography is the best method for identifying gallbladder stones and for confirming extrahepatic biliary obstruction as dilated bile ducts are visible. It is good at identifying liver abnormalities such as cysts and tumours and pancreatic masses and fluid collections, but visualisation of the lower common bile duct and pancreas is often hindered by overlying bowel gas. Computed tomography is complementary to ultrasonography and provides information on liver texture, gallbladder disease, bile duct dilatation, and pancreatic disease. Computed tomography is particularly valuable for detecting small lesions in the liver and pancreas.

Cholangiography identifies the level of biliary obstruction and often the cause. Intravenous cholangiography is rarely used now as opacification of the bile ducts is poor, particularly in jaundiced patients, and anaphylaxis remains a problem. Endoscopic retrograde cholangiopancreatography is advisable when the lower end of the duct is obstructed (by gall stones or carcinoma of the pancreas). The cause of the obstruction (for example, stones or parasites) can sometimes be removed by endoscopic retrograde cholangiopancreatography to allow cytological or histological diagnosis.

Percutaneous transhepatic cholangiography is preferred for hilar obstructions (biliary stricture, cholangiocarcinoma of the hepatic duct bifurcation) because better opacification of the ducts near the obstruction provides more information for planning subsequent management. Obstruction can be relieved by insertion of a plastic or metal tube (a stent) at either endoscopic retrograde cholangiopancreatography or percutaneous transhepatic cholangiography.

Magnetic resonance cholangiopancreatography allows non-invasive visualisation of the bile and pancreatic ducts. It is

> **Ultrasonography is the most useful initial investigation in patients with jaundice**

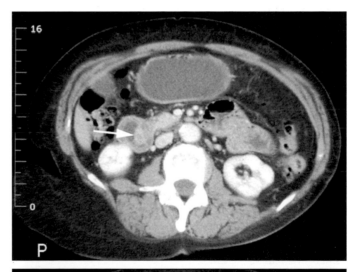

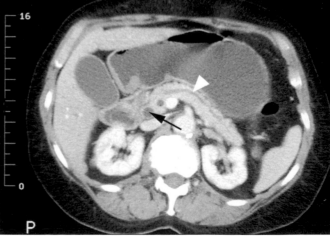

Figure 1.3 Computed tomogram of ampullary carcinoma (white arrow) causing obstruction of the bile duct (black arrow, bottom) and pancreatic ducts (white arrowhead)

superseding most diagnostic endoscopic cholangiopancreatography as faster magnetic resonance imaging scanners become more widely available.

Liver biopsy

Percutaneous liver biopsy is a day case procedure performed under local anaesthetic. Patients must have a normal clotting time and platelet count and ultrasonography to ensure that the bile ducts are not dilated. Complications include bile leaks and haemorrhage, and overall mortality is around 0.1%. A transjugular liver biopsy can be performed by passing a special needle, under radiological guidance, through the internal jugular vein, the right atrium, and inferior vena cava and into the liver though the hepatic veins. This has the advantage that clotting time does not need to be normal as bleeding from the liver is not a problem. Liver biopsy is essential to diagnose chronic hepatitis and establish the cause of cirrhosis.

Ultrasound guided liver biopsy can be used to diagnose liver masses. However, it may cause bleeding (especially with liver cell adenomas), anaphylactic shock (hydatid cysts), or tumour seeding (hepatocellular carcinoma or metastases). Many lesions can be confidently diagnosed by using a combination of imaging methods (ultrasonography, spiral computed tomography, magnetic resonance imaging, nuclear medicine, laparoscopy, and laparoscopic ultrasonography). When malignancy is suspected in solitary lesions or those confined to one half of the liver, resection is the best way to avoid compromising a potentially curative procedure.

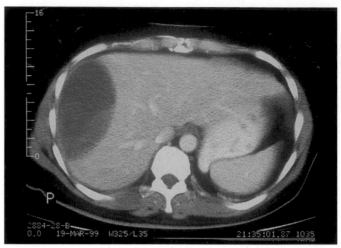

Figure 1.4 Subcapsular haematoma: a complication of liver biopsy

---

Summary points

- An isolated raised serum bilirubin concentration is usually due to Gilbert's syndrome, which is confirmed by normal liver enzyme activities and full blood count
- Jaundice with dark urine, pale stools, and raised alkaline phosphatase and γ-glutamyl transferase activity suggests an obstructive cause, which is confirmed by presence of dilated bile ducts on ultrasonography
- Jaundice in patients with low serum albumin concentration suggests chronic liver disease
- Patients with high concentrations of bilirubin (> 100 μmol/l) or signs of sepsis require emergency specialist referral
- Imaging of the bile ducts for obstructive jaundice is increasingly performed by magnetic resonance cholangiopancreatography, with endoscopy becoming reserved for therapeutic interventions

---

2 Gallstone disease

I J Beckingham

Gall stones are the most common abdominal reason for admission to hospital in developed countries and account for an important part of healthcare expenditure. Around 5.5 million people have gall stones in the United Kingdom, and over 50 000 cholecystectomies are performed each year.

Types of gall stone and aetiology

Normal bile consists of 70% bile salts (mainly cholic and chenodeoxycholic acids), 22% phospholipids (lecithin), 4% cholesterol, 3% proteins, and 0.3% bilirubin. Cholesterol or cholesterol predominant (mixed) stones account for 80% of all gall stones in the United Kingdom and form when there is supersaturation of bile with cholesterol. Formation of stones is further aided by decreased gallbladder motility. Black pigment stones consist of 70% calcium bilirubinate and are more common in patients with haemolytic diseases (sickle cell anaemia, hereditary spherocytosis, thalassaemia) and cirrhosis.

Brown pigment stones are uncommon in Britain (accounting for <5% of stones) and are formed within the intrahepatic and extrahepatic bile ducts as well as the gall bladder. They form as a result of stasis and infection within the biliary system, usually in the presence of *Escherichia coli* and *Klebsiella spp,* which produce β glucuronidase that converts soluble conjugated bilirubin back to the insoluble unconjugated state leading to the formation of soft, earthy, brown stones. *Ascaris lumbricoides* and *Opisthorchis senensis* have both been implicated in the formation of these stones, which are common in South East Asia.

Clinical presentations

Biliary colic or chronic cholecystitis
The commonest presentation of gallstone disease is biliary pain. The pain starts suddenly in the epigastrium or right upper quadrant and may radiate round to the back in the interscapular region. Contrary to its name, the pain often does not fluctuate but persists from 15 minutes up to 24 hours, subsiding spontaneously or with opioid analgesics. Nausea or vomiting often accompanies the pain, which is visceral in origin and occurs as a result of distension of the gallbladder due to an obstruction or to the passage of a stone through the cystic duct.

Most episodes can be managed at home with analgesics and antiemetics. Pain continuing for over 24 hours or accompanied by fever suggests acute cholecystitis and usually necessitates hospital admission. Ultrasonography is the definitive investigation for gall stones. It has a 95% sensitivity and specificity for stones over 4 mm in diameter.

Non-specific abdominal pain, early satiety, fat intolerance, nausea, and bowel symptoms occur with comparable frequency in patients with and without gall stones, and these symptoms respond poorly to inappropriate cholecystectomy. In many of these patients symptoms are due to upper gastrointestinal tract problems or irritable bowel syndrome.

Acute cholecystitis
When obstruction of the cystic duct persists, an acute inflammatory response may develop with a leucocytosis and mild fever. Irritation of the adjacent parietal peritoneum causes

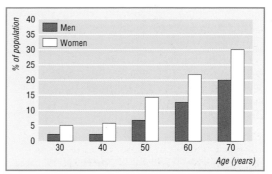

Figure 2.1 Prevalence of gall stones in United Kingdom according to age

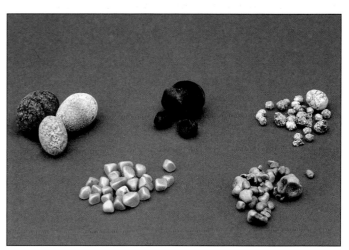

Figure 2.2 Gall stones vary from pure cholesterol (white), through mixed, to bile salt predominant (black)

Box 1.1 Risk factors associated with formation of cholesterol gall stones
- Age >40 years
- Female sex (twice risk in men)
- Genetic or ethnic variation
- High fat, low fibre diet
- Obesity
- Pregnancy (risk increases with number of pregnancies)
- Hyperlipidaemia
- Bile salt loss (ileal disease or resection)
- Diabetes mellitus
- Cystic fibrosis
- Antihyperlipidaemic drugs (clofibrate)
- Gallbladder dysmotility
- Prolonged fasting
- Total parenteral nutrition

Box 1.2 Differential diagnosis of common causes of severe acute epigastric pain
- Biliary colic
- Peptic ulcer disease
- Oesophageal spasm
- Myocardial infarction
- Acute pancreatitis

---

localised tenderness in the right upper quadrant. As well as gall stones, ultrasonography may show a tender, thick walled, oedematous gall bladder with an abnormal amount of adjacent fluid. Liver enzyme activities are often mildly abnormal.

Initial management is with non-steroidal anti-inflammatory drugs (intramuscular or per rectum) or opioid analgesic. Although acute cholecystitis is initially a chemical inflammation, secondary bacterial infection is common, and patients should be given a broad spectrum parenteral antibiotic (such as a second generation cephalosporin).

Progress is monitored by resolution of tachycardia, fever, and tenderness. Ideally cholecystectomy should be performed during the same admission as delayed cholecystectomy has a 15% failure rate (empyema, gangrene, or perforation) and a 15% readmission rate with further pain.

Jaundice

Jaundice occurs in patients with gall stones when a stone migrates from the gall bladder into the common bile duct or, less commonly, when fibrosis and impaction of a large stone in Hartmann's pouch compresses the common hepatic duct (Mirrizi's syndrome). Liver function tests show a cholestatic pattern (raised conjugated bilirubin concentration and alkaline phosphatase activity with normal or mildly raised aspartate transaminase activity) and ultrasonography confirms dilatation of the common bile duct (>7 mm diameter) usually without distention of the gall bladder.

Acute cholangitis

When an obstructed common bile duct becomes contaminated with bacteria, usually from the duodenum, cholangitis may develop. Urgent treatment is required with broad spectrum antibiotics together with early decompression of the biliary system by endoscopic or radiological stenting or surgical drainage if stenting is not available. Delay may result in septicaemia or the development of liver abscesses, which are associated with a high mortality.

Acute pancreatitis

Acute pancreatitis develops in 5% of all patients with gall stones and is more common in patients with multiple small stones, a wide cystic duct, and a common channel between the common bile duct and pancreatic duct. Small stones passing down the common bile duct and through the papilla may temporarily obstruct the pancreatic duct or allow reflux of duodenal fluid or bile into the pancreatic duct resulting in acute pancreatitis. Patients should be given intravenous fluids and analgesia and be monitored carefully for the development of organ failure (see later article on acute pancreatitis).

Gallstone ileus

Acute cholecystitis may cause the gall bladder to adhere to the adjacent jejunum or duodenum. Subsequent inflammation may result in a fistula between these structures and the passage of a gall stone into the bowel. Large stones may become impacted and obstruct the small bowel. Abdominal radiography shows obstruction of the small bowel and air in the biliary tree. Treatment is by laparotomy and "milking" the obstructing stone into the colon or by enterotomy and extraction.

Natural course of gallstone disease

Two thirds of gall stones are asymptomatic, and the yearly risk of developing biliary pain is 1-4%. Patients with asymptomatic gall stones seldom develop complications. Prophylactic cholecystectomy is therefore not recommended when stones

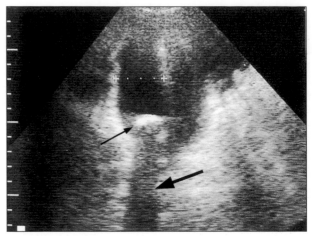

Figure 2.3 Ultrasonogram showing large gall stone (thin arrow) casting acoustic shadow (thick arrow) in gall bladder

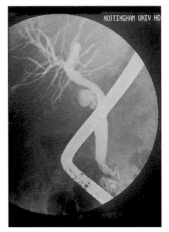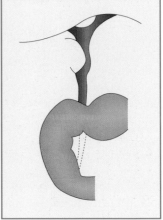

Figure 2.4 Type 1 Mirrizi's syndrome: gallbladder stone in Hartmann's pouch compressing common bile duct and causing deranged liver function

---

Box 1.3 Charcot's triad of symptoms in severe cholangitis
- Pain in right upper quadrant
- Jaundice
- High swinging fever with rigors and chills

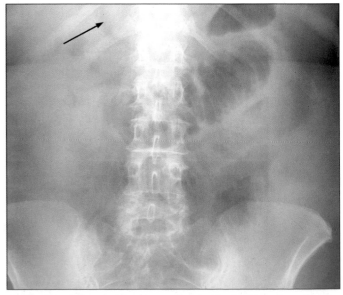

Figure 2.5 Small bowel obstruction and gas in bile ducts in patient with gallstone ileus

are discovered incidentally by radiography or ultrasonography during the investigation of other symptoms. Although gall stones are associated with cancer of the gall bladder, the risk of developing cancer in patients with asymptomatic gall stones is <0.01%—less than the mortality associated with cholecystectomy.

Patients with symptomatic gall stones have an annual rate of developing complications of 1-2% and a 50% chance of a further episode of biliary colic. They should be offered treatment.

Management of gallstone disease

Cholecystectomy

Cholecystectomy is the optimal management as it removes both the gall stones and the gall bladder, preventing recurrent disease. The only common consequence of removing the gall bladder is an increase in stool frequency, which is clinically important in less than 5% of patients and responds well to standard antidiarrhoeal drugs when necessary.

Laparoscopic cholecystectomy has been adopted rapidly since its introduction in 1987, and 80-90% of cholecystectomies in the United Kingdom are now carried out in this way. The only specific contraindications to laparoscopic cholecystectomy are coagulopathy and the later stages of pregnancy. Acute cholecystitis and previous gastroduodenal surgery are no longer contraindications but are associated with a higher rate of conversion to open cholecystectomy.

Laparoscopic cholecystectomy has a lower mortality than the standard open procedure (0.1% v 0.5% for the open procedure). This is mainly because of a lower incidence of postoperative cardiac and respiratory complications. The smaller incisions cause less pain, which reduces the requirement for opioid analgesics. Patients usually stay in hospital for only one night in most centres, and the procedure can be done as a day case in selected patients. Most patients are able to return to sedentary work after 7-10 days. This decrease in overall morbidity and earlier recovery has led to a 25% increase in the rate of cholecystectomy in some countries.

The main disadvantage of the laparoscopic technique has been a higher incidence of injury to the common hepatic or bile ducts (0.2-0.4% v 0.1% for open cholecystectomy). Higher rates of injury are associated with inexperienced surgeons (the "learning curve" phenomenon) and acute cholecystitis. Furthermore, injuries to the common bile duct tend to be more extensive with laparoscopic surgery. However, there is some evidence suggesting that the rates of injury are now falling.

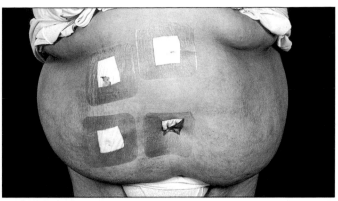

Figure 2.6 Laparoscopic cholecystectomy reduces the risk of surgery in morbidly obese patients

---

Box 1.4 Causes of pain after cholecystectomy
- Retained or recurrent stone (dilatation of common bile duct seen in only 30% of patients)
- Iatrogenic biliary leak or stricture of common bile duct
- Papillary stenosis or dysfunctional sphincter of Oddi
- Incorrect preoperative diagnosis—for example, irritable bowel syndrome, peptic ulcer, gastro-oesophageal reflux

---

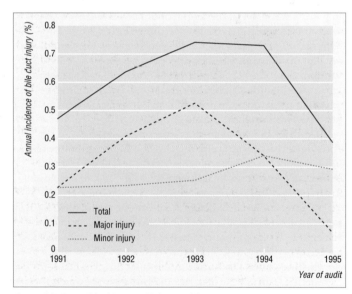

Figure 2.7 Annual incidence of injury to bile duct during laparoscopic cholescystectomy, United Kingdom,1991-5. Adapted from *Br J Surg* 1996;83:1356-60

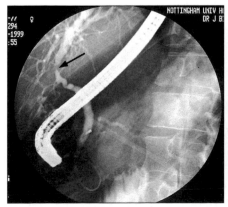
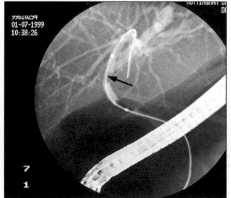
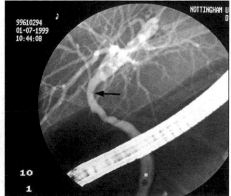

Figure 2.8 Injury to common bile duct incurred during laparoscopic cholecystectomy before, during, and after repair by balloon dilatation

Alternative treatments

Several non-surgical techniques have been used to treat gall stones including oral dissolution therapy (chenodeoxycholic and ursodeoxycholic acid), contact dissolution (direct instillation of methyltetrabutyl ether or mono-octanoin), and stone shattering with extracorporeal shockwave lithotripsy.

Less than 10% of gall stones are suitable for non-surgical treatment, and success rates vary widely. Stones are cleared in around half of appropriately selected patients. In addition, patients require expensive, lifelong treatment to counteract bile acid in order to prevent stones from reforming. These treatments should be used only in patients who refuse surgery.

Managing common bile duct stones

Around 10% of patients with stones in the gallbladder have stones in the common bile duct. Patients may present with jaundice or acute pancreatitis; the results of liver function tests are characteristic of cholestasis and a dilated common bile duct is visible on ultrasonography.

The optimal treatment is to remove the stones in both the common bile duct and the gall bladder. This can be performed in two stages by endocsopic retrograde cholangiopancreatography followed by laparoscopic cholecystectomy or as a single stage cholecystectomy with exploration of the common bile duct by laparoscopic or open surgery. The morbidity and mortality (2%) of open surgery is higher than for the laparoscopic option. Two recent randomised controlled trials have shown laparoscopic exploration of the bile duct to be as effective as endoscopic retrograde cholangiopancreatography in removing stones from the common bile duct. Laparoscopic exploration has the advantage that the gall bladder is removed in a single stage procedure, thus reducing hospital stay. In practice, management often depends on local availability and skills.

In elderly or frail patients endoscopic retrograde cholangiopancreatography with division of the sphincter of Oddi (sphincterotomy) and stone extraction alone (without cholecsytectomy) may be appropriate as the risk of developing further symptoms is only 10% in this population.

When stones in the common bile duct are suspected in patients who have had a cholecystectomy, endoscopic retrograde cholangiopancreatography can be used to diagnose and remove the stones. Stones are removed with the aid of a dormia basket or balloon. For multiple stones, a pigtail stent can be inserted to drain the bile; this often allows subsequent passage of the stones. Large or hard stones can be crushed with a mechanical lithotripter. When cholangiopancreatography is not technically possible the stones have to be removed surgically.

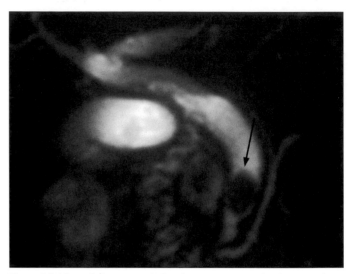

Figure 2.9 Magnetic resonance cholangiopancreatogram showing stone in common bile duct

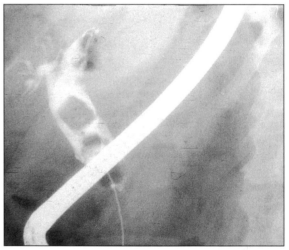

Figure 2.10p Large angular common bile duct stones. These are difficult to remove endoscopically

Further reading
- Beckingham IJ, Rowlands BJ. Post cholecystectomy problems. In Blumgart H, ed. *Surgery of the liver and biliary tract.* 3rd ed. London: WB Saunders, 2000
- National Institutes of Health consensus development conference statement on gallstones and laparoscopic cholecystectomy *Am J Surg* 1993;165:390-8
- Cuschieri A, Lezoche E, Morino M, Croce E, Lacy A, Toouli J, et al. EAES multicenter prospective randomized trial comparing two-stage vs single-stage management of patients with gallstone disease and ductal calculi. *Surg Endosc* 1999;13:952-7

Summary points
- Gall stones are the commonest cause for emergency hospital admission with abdominal pain
- Laparoscopic cholecystectomy has become the treatment of choice for gallbladder stones
- Risk of bile duct injury with laparoscopic cholecystectomy is around 0.2%
- Asymptomatic gall stones do not require treatment
- Cholangitis requires urgent treatment with antibiotics and biliary decompression by endoscopic retrograde cholangiopancreatography

3 Acute hepatitis

S D Ryder, I J Beckingham

Acute hepatic injury is confirmed by a raised serum alanine transaminase activity. The activity may be 100 times normal, and no other biochemical test has been shown to be a better indicator. Alkaline phosphatase and γ-glutamyltransferase activities can also be raised in patients with an acute hepatic injury, but their activites are usually proportionately lower than that of alanine transaminase.

Table 3.1 Liver enzyme activity in liver disease

	Hepatitis	Cholestasis or obstruction	"Mixed"
Alkaline phosphatase	Normal	Raised	Raised
γ-glutamyltransferase	Normal	Raised	Raised
Alanine transaminase	Raised	Normal	Raised

Acute viral hepatitis

Hepatitis can be caused by the hepatitis viruses A, B, C, D, or E. The D and E forms are rare in the United Kingdom. A large proportion of infections with hepatitis viruses of all types are asymptomatic or result in anicteric illnesses that may not be diagnosed as hepatitis. Hepatitis A virus causes a typically minor illness in childhood, with more than 80% of cases being asymptomatic. In adult life infection is more likely to produce clinical symptoms, although only a third of patients with acute hepatitis A infections are jaundiced. Infections with hepatitis B and C viruses are also usually asymptomatic except in intravenous drug users, in whom 30% of hepatitis B infections are associated with jaundice.

In the preicteric phase, patients often have non-specific systemic symptoms together with discomfort in the right upper quadrant of the abdomen. An illness resembling serum sickness occurs in about 10% of patients with acute hepatitis B infection and 5-10% of patients with acute hepatitis C infection. This presents with a maculopapular rash and arthralgia, typically affecting the wrist, knees, elbows, and ankles. It is due to formation of immune complexes, and patients often test positive for rheumatoid factor. It is almost always self limiting, and usually settles rapidly after the onset of jaundice.

Rarely, patients with acute hepatitis B infection present with acute pancreatitis. Up to 30% of patients have raised amylase activity, and postmortem examinations in patients with fulminant hepatitis B show histological changes of pancreatitis in up to 50%. Myocarditis, pericarditis, pleural effusion, aplastic anaemia, encephalitis, and polyneuritis have all been reported in patients with hepatitis.

Box 3.1 Common symptoms of acute viral hepatitis

- Myalgia
- Nausea and vomiting
- Fatigue and malaise
- Change in sense of smell or taste
- Right upper abdominal pain
- Coryza, photophobia, headache
- Diarrhoea (may have pale stools and dark urine)

Table 3.2 Types and modes of transmission of human hepatitis viruses

	A	B	C	D	E
Virus type	Picorna-viridae	Hepadna-viridae	Flavi-viridae	Delta-viridae	Calci-viridae
Nucleic acid	RNA	DNA	RNA	RNA	RNA
Mean (range) incubation period (days)	30 (15-50)	80 (28-160)	50 (14-160)	Variable	40 (15-45)
Mode of transmission:					
Orofaecal	Yes	Possible	No	No	Yes
Sexual	Yes	Yes	Rare	Yes	No
Blood	Rare	Yes	Yes	Yes	No
Chronic infection	No	Yes	Yes	Yes	No

Physical signs in viral hepatitis

Physical examination of patients before the development of jaundice usually shows no abnormality, although hepatomegaly (10% of patients), splenomegaly (5%), and lymphadenopathy (5%) may be present. Patients with an acute illness should not have signs of chronic liver disease. The presence of these signs suggests that the illness is either the direct result of chronic liver disease or that the patient has an acute event superimposed on a background of chronic liver disease—for example, hepatitis D virus superinfection in a carrier of hepatitis B virus.

A small proportion of patients with acute viral hepatitis develop a profound cholestatic illness. This is most common with hepatitis A and can be prolonged, with occasional patients remaining jaundiced for up to eight months.

Box 3.2 Other biochemical or haematological abnormalities seen in acute hepatitis

- Leucopenia is common ($<5 \times 10^9$/l in 10% of patients)
- Anaemia and thrombocytopenia
- Immunoglobulin titres may be raised

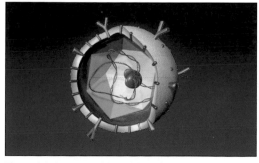

Figure 3.1 Structure of hepatitis B virus

Acute liver failure (fulminant hepatitis)

Death from acute viral hepatitis is usually due to the development of fulminant hepatitis. This is usually defined as development of hepatic encephalopathy within eight weeks of symptoms or within two weeks of onset of jaundice. The risk of developing fulminant liver failure is generally low, but there are groups with higher risks. Pregnant women with acute hepatitis E infection have a risk of fulminant liver failure of around 15% with a mortality of 5%. The risk of developing fulminant liver failure in hepatitis A infection increases with age and with pre-existing liver disease. Fulminant hepatitis B is seen in adult infection and is relatively rare.

The primary clinical features of acute liver failure are encephalopathy and jaundice. Jaundice almost always precedes encephalopathy in acute liver failure The peak of alanine transaminase activity does not correlate with the risk of developing liver failure. Prolonged coagulation is the biochemical hallmark of liver failure and is due to lack of synthesis of liver derived factors. Prolongation of the prothrombin time in acute hepatitis, even if the patient is clinically well without signs of encephalopathy, should be regarded as sinister and the patient monitored closely. Hypoglycaemia is seen only in fulminant liver disease and can be severe.

Diagnosis of acute hepatitis

Hepatitis A
Hepatitis A infection can be reliably diagnosed by the presence of antihepatitis A IgM. This test has high sensitivity and specificity. Occasional false positive results occur in patients with liver disease due to other causes if high titres of immunoglobulin are present, but the clinical context usually makes this obvious.

Hepatitis B
Hepatitis B infection is usually characterised by the presence of hepatitis B surface antigen. Other markers are used to determine if the virus is active and replicating, when it can cause serious liver damage.

In acute hepatitis B infection the serology can be difficult to interpret. Acute hepatitis develops because of immune recognition of infected liver cells, which results in T cell mediated killing of hepatocytes. Active regeneration of hepatocytes then occurs. As well as a cell mediated immune response, a humoral immune response develops; this is probably important in removing viral particles from the blood and thus preventing reinfection of hepatocytes. Because of the immune response attempting to eradicate hepatitis B virus, viral replication may already have ceased by the time a patient presents with acute hepatitis B, and the patient may be positive for hepatitis B surface antigen and negative for e antigen.

It is difficult in this situation to be certain that the patient had acute hepatitis B and that the serology does not imply past infection unrelated to the current episode. To enable a clear diagnosis, most reference centres now report the titre of IgM antibody to hepatitis B core antigen (IgM anticore). As core antigen never appears in serum, its presence implies an immune response against hepatitis B virus within liver cells and is a sensitive and specific marker of acute hepatitis B infection.

Rarely, the immune response to hepatitis B infection is so rapid that even hepatitis B surface antigen has been cleared from the serum by the time of presentation with jaundice. This may be more common in patients developing severe acute liver disease and has been reported in up to 5% of patients with fulminant hepatitis diagnosed by an appropriate pattern of antibody response.

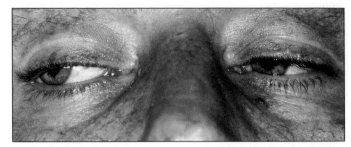

Figure 3.2 Disconjugate gaze due to cerebral oedema in jaundiced patient with fulminant hepatitis

> **The onset of confusion or drowsiness in a patient with acute viral hepatitis is always sinister**

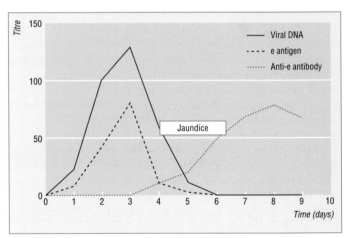

Figure 3.3 Appearance of serological markers in acute self limiting hepatitis B virus infection

> **Replication of hepatitis B virus is assessed by measuring e antigen (a truncated version of the hepatitis B core antigen that contains the viral replication mechanism) and hepatitis B DNA**

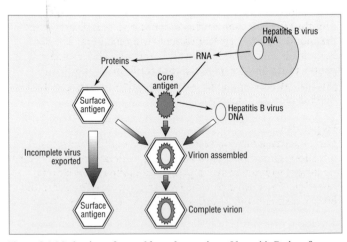

Figure 3.4 Mechanism of assembly and excretion of hepatitis B virus from infected hepatocytes

Hepatitis C

Screening tests for hepatitis C virus infection use enzyme linked immunosorbent assays (ELISA) with recombinant viral antigens on patients' serum. Acute hepatitis C cannot be reliably diagnosed by antibody tests as these often do not give positive results for up to three months.

Hepatitis C virus was the cause of more than 90% of all post-transfusion hepatitis in Europe and the United States. Before 1991, the risk of infection in the United Kingdom was 0.2% per unit of blood transfused, but this has fallen to 1 infection per 10 000 units transfused since the introduction of routine serological screening of blood donors. Acute hepatitis C infection is therefore now seen commonly only in intravenous drug users.

Antibodies to hepatitis C appear relatively late in the course of the infection, and if clinical suspicion is high, the patient's serum should be tested for hepatitis C virus RNA to establish the diagnosis.

Non-A-E viral hepatitis

Epstein Barr virus causes rises in liver enzyme activities in almost all cases of acute infection, but it is uncommon for the liver injury to be sufficiently severe to cause jaundice. When jaundice does occur in patients with Epstein Barr virus infection, it can be prolonged with a large cholestatic element. Diagnosis is usually relatively easy because the typical symptoms of Epstein Barr infection are almost always present and serological testing usually gives positive results. Cytomegalovirus can also cause acute hepatitis. This is unusual, rarely severe, and runs a chronic course only in immunosuppressed patients.

The cause of about 7% of all episodes of acute presumed viral hepatitis remains unidentified. It seems certain that other viral agents will be identified that cause acute liver injury.

Management of acute viral hepatitis

Hepatitis A

Most patients with hepatitis A infection have a self limiting illness that will settle totally within a few weeks. Management is conservative, with tests being aimed at identifying the small group of patients at risk of developing fulminant liver failure.

Hepatitis B

Acute hepatitis B is also usually self limiting, and most patients who contract the virus will clear it completely. All cases must be notified and sexual and close household contacts screened and vaccinated. Patients should be monitored to ensure fulminant liver failure does not develop and have serological testing three months after infection to check that the virus is cleared from the blood. About 5-10% of patients will remain positive for hepatitis B surface antigen at three months, and a smaller proportion will have ongoing viral replication (e antigen positive). All such patients require expert follow up (see article on chronic viral hepatitis).

Hepatitis C

Early identification and referral of cases of acute hepatitis C infection is important because strong evidence exists that early treatment with interferon alpha reduces the risk of chronic infection. The rate of chronicity in untreated patients is about 80%; treatment with interferon reduces this to below 50%.

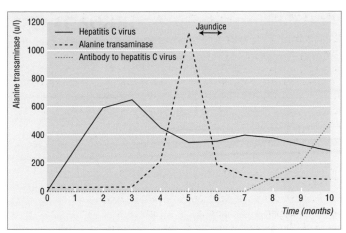

Figure 3.5 Appearance of hepatitis C virus RNA, antibodies to hepatitis C virus, and raised alanine transaminase activity in acute hepatitis C infection

---

Box 3.3 Hepatitis D and E infection

Hepatitis D
- Incomplete RNA virus that requires hepatitis B surface antigen to transmit its genome from cell to cell
- Occurs only in patients positive for hepatitis B surface antigen
- Usually confined to intravenous drug users in United Kingdom

Hepatitis E
- Transmitted by orofaecal route
- Produces an acute self limiting illness similar to hepatitis A
- Common in developing world
- High mortality in pregnant women

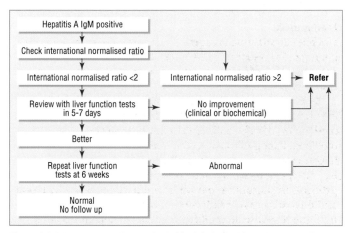

Figure 3.6 Management of acute hepatitis A infection in general practice

---

Summary points

- Symptoms of hepatitis are non-specific and often occur without the development of jaundice
- Serum alanine transaminase is the most useful screening test for hepatitis in general practice
- Hepatitis A rarely causes fulminant liver failure or chronic liver disease
- In the developed world, new cases of hepatitis C are mainly seen in intravenous drug users
- Most adults who contract hepatitis B virus clear the virus, with < 10% developing chronic liver infection

4   Chronic viral hepatitis

S D Ryder, I J Beckingham

Most cases of chronic viral hepatitis are caused by hepatitis B or C virus. Hepatitis B virus is one of the commonest chronic viral infections in the world, with about 170 million people chronically infected worldwide. In developed countries it is relatively uncommon, with a prevalence of 1 per 550 population in the United Kingdom and United States.

The main method of spread in areas of high endemicity is vertical transmission from carrier mother to child, and this may account for 40-50% of all hepatitis B infections in such areas. Vertical transmission is highly efficient; more than 95% of children born to infected mothers become infected and develop chronic viral infection. In low endemicity countries, the virus is mainly spread by sexual or blood contact among people at high risk, including intravenous drug users, patients receiving haemodialysis, homosexual men, and people living in institutions, especially those with learning disabilities. These high risk groups are much less likely to develop chronic viral infection (5-10%). Men are more likely then women to develop chronic infection, although the reasons for this are unclear.

Up to 300 million people have chronic hepatitis C infection mainly worldwide. Unlike hepatitis B virus, hepatitis C infection is not mainly confined to the developing world, with 0.3% to 0.7% of the United Kingdom population infected. The virus is spread almost exclusively by blood contact. About 15% of infected patients in Northern Europe have a history of blood transfusion and about 70% have used intravenous drugs. Sexual transmission does occur, but is unusual; less than 5% of long term sexual partners become infected. Vertical transmission is also unusual.

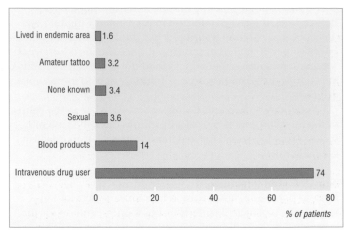

Figure 4.1 Risk factors for hepatitis C virus infection among 1500 patients in Trent region,1998. Note: professional tattooing does not carry a risk

Presentation

Chronic viral liver disease may be detected as a result of finding abnormal liver biochemistry during serological testing of asymptomatic patients in high risk groups or as a result of the complications of cirrhosis. Patients with chronic viral hepatitis usually have a sustained increase in alanine transaminase activity. The rise is lower than in acute infection, usually only two or three times the upper limit of normal. In hepatitis C infection, the γ-glutamyltransferase activity is also often raised. The degree of the rise in transaminase activity has little relevance to the extent of underlying hepatic inflammation. This is particularly true of hepatitis C infection, when patients often have normal transaminase activity despite active liver inflammation.

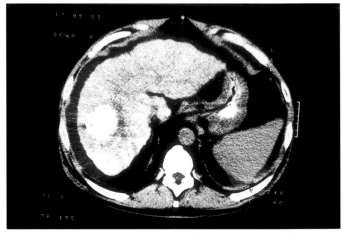

Figure 4.2 Computed tomogram showing hepatocellular carcinoma, a common complication of cirrhosis

Hepatitis B

Most patients with chronic hepatitis B infection will be positive for hepatitis B surface antigen. Hepatitis B surface antigen is on the viral coat, and its presence in blood implies that the patient is infected. Measurement of viral DNA in blood has replaced e antigen as the most sensitive measure of viral activity.

Chronic hepatitis B virus infection can be thought of as occurring in phases dependent on the degree of immune response to the virus. If a person is infected when the immune response is "immature," there is little or no response to the hepatitis B virus. The concentrations of hepatitis B viral DNA in serum are very high, the hepatocytes contain abundant viral

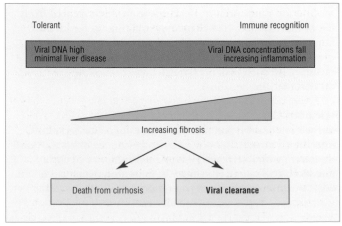

Figure 4.3 Phases of infection with hepatitis B virus

particles (surface antigen and core antigen) but little or no ongoing hepatocyte death is seen on liver biopsy because of the defective immune response. Over some years the degree of immune recognition usually increases. At this stage the concentration of viral DNA tends to fall and liver biopsy shows increasing inflammation in the liver. Two outcomes are then possible, either the immune response is adequate and the virus is inactivated and removed from the system or the attempt at removal results in extensive fibrosis, distortion of the normal liver architecture, and eventually death from the complications of cirrhosis.

Assessment of chronic hepatitis B infection

Patients positive for hepatitis B surface antigen with no evidence of viral replication, normal liver enzyme activity, and normal appearance on liver ultrasonography require no further investigation. Such patients have a low risk of developing symptomatic liver disease or hepatocellular carcinoma. Reactivation of B virus replication can occur, and patients should therefore have yearly serological and liver enzyme tests.

Patients with abnormal liver biochemistry, even without detectable hepatitis B viral DNA or an abnormal liver texture on ultrasonography, should have liver biopsy, as 5% of patients with only surface antigen carriage at presentation will have cirrhosis. Detection of cirrhosis is important as patients are at risk of complications, including variceal bleeding and hepatocellular carcinoma. Patients with repeatedly normal alanine transaminase activity and high concentrations of viral DNA are extremely unlikely to have developed advanced liver disease, and biopsy is not always required at this stage.

Treatment

Interferon alfa was first shown to be effective for some patients with hepatitis B infection in the 1980s, and it remains the mainstay of treatment. The optimal dose and duration of interferon for hepatitis B is somewhat contentious, but most clinicians use 8-10 million units three times a week for four to six months. Overall, the probability of response (that is, stopping viral replication) to interferon therapy is around 40%. Few patients lose all markers of infection with hepatitis B, and surface antigen usually remains in the serum. Successful treatment with interferon produces a sustained improvement in liver histology and reduces the risk of developing end stage liver disease. The risk of hepatocellular carcinoma is also probably reduced but is not abolished in those who remain positive for hepatitis B surface antigen.

In general, about 15% of patients receiving interferon have no side effects, 15% cannot tolerate treatment, and the remaining 70% experience side effects but are able to continue treatment. Depression can be a serious problem, and both suicide and admissions with acute psychosis are well described. Viral clearance occurs through induction of immune mediated killing of infected hepatocytes. Transient hepatitis can therefore occasionally cause severe decompensation requiring liver transplantation.

Lamivudine is a nucleoside analogue that is a potent inhibitor of hepatitis B viral DNA replication. It has a good safety profile and has been widely tested in patients with chronic hepatitis B virus infection, mainly in the Far East. In long term trials almost all treated patients showed prompt and sustained inhibition of viral DNA replication, with about 17% becoming e antigen negative when treatment was continued for 12 months. There was an associated improvement of inflammation and a reduction in progression of fibrosis on liver biopsy. Side effects are generally mild. Combination therapy with interferon and lamivudine has not been found to have additional benefit.

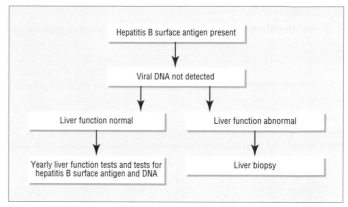

Figure 4.4 Investigation of patients positive for hepatitis B surface antigen without viral replication

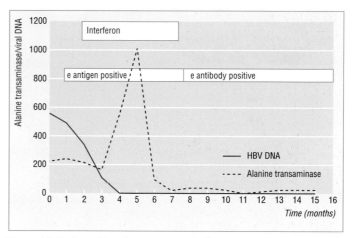

Figure 4.5 Timing of interferon treatment in the management of hepatitis B

Table 4.1 Factors indicating likelihood of response to interferon in chronic hepatitis B infection

	High probability	Low probablility
Age (years)	<50	>50
Sex	Female	Male
Viral DNA	Low	High
Activity of liver inflammation	High	Low
Country of origin ·	Western world	Asia or Africa
Coinfection with HIV	Absent	Present

Table 4.2 Side effects of treatment with interferon alpha

Symptoms	Frequency (%)
Fever or flu-like illness	80
Depression	25
Fatigue	50
Haematological abnormalities	10
No side effects	15

Hepatitis C

Chronic hepatitis C virus infection has a long course, and most patients are diagnosed in a presymptomatic stage. In the United Kingdom, most patients are now discovered because of an identifiable risk factor (intravenous drug use, family history, or blood transfusion) or because of abnormal liver biochemistry. Screening for hepatitis C virus infection is based on enzyme linked immmonosorbent assays (ELISA) using recombinant viral antigens and patients' serum. These have high sensitivity and specificity. The diagnosis is confirmed by radioimmunoblot and direct detection of viral RNA in peripheral blood by polymerase chain reaction. Viral RNA is regarded as the best test to determine infectivity and assess response to treatment.

Natural course of hepatitis C infection

In order to assess the need for treatment it is important to have a clear understanding of the natural course of hepatitis C infection and factors that may predispose to more severe outcome. Our knowledge is limited because of the relatively recent discovery of the virus. It is clear, however, that hepatitis C is usually slowly progressive, with an average time from infection to development of cirrhosis of around 30 years, albeit with a high level of variability. The main factors associated with increased risk of progressive liver disease are age >40 at infection, high alcohol consumption, and male sex.

Viraemic patients with abnormal alanine transaminase activity need a liver biopsy to assess the stage of disease (amount of fibrosis) and degree of necroinflammatory change (Knodell score). Management is usually based on the degree of liver damage, with patients with more severe disease being offered treatment. Patients with mild changes are usually followed up without treatment as their prognosis is good and future treatment is likely to be more effective than present regimens.

Treatment of hepatitis C

Interferon alfa (3 million units three times a week) in combination with tribavirin (1000 mg a day for patients under 75 kg and 1200 mg for patients $\geqslant$75 kg) has recently been shown to be more effective than interferon alone. A large study in Europe showed no advantage to continuing treatment beyond six months in patients who had a good chance of response, whereas those with a poorer outlook needed longer treatment (12 months) to maximise the chance of clearing their infection. About 30% of patients will obtain a "cure" (sustained response). The main determinant of response is viral genotype, with genotypes 1 and 4 having poor response rates.

Combination therapy has the same side effects as interferon monotherapy with the additional risk of haemolytic anaemia. Patients developing anaemia should have their dose of tribavirin reduced. All patients should have a full blood count and liver function tests weekly for the first four weeks of treatment and monthly thereafter if haemoglobin concentration and white cell count are stable. Many new treatments are currently entering clinical trials, including long acting interferons and alternative antiviral drugs.

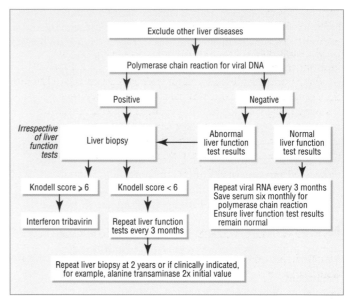

Figure 4.6 Management of chronic hepatitis C virus infection

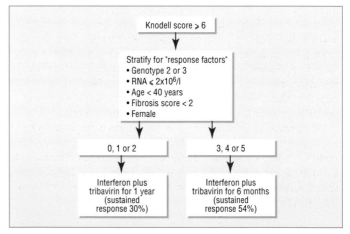

Figure 4.7 Combination therapy for hepatitis C

Summary points
- Viral hepatitis is relatively common in United Kingdom (mainly hepatitis C)
- Presentation is usually with abnormal alanine transaminase activity
- Disease progression in hepatitis C is usually slow (median time to development of cirrhosis around 30 years)
- Liver biopsy is essential in managing chronic viral hepatitis
- New treatments for hepatitis C (interferon and tribavirin) and hepatitis B (lamivudine) have improved the chances of eliminating these pathogens from chronically infected patients

Further reading
Szmuness W. Hepatocellular carcinoma and the hepatitis B virus: evidence for a causal association. *Prog Med Virol* 1978;24:40-8.
Stevens CE, Beasley RP, Tsui V, Lee WC. Vertical transmission of hepatitis B antigen in Taiwan. *N Engl J Med* 1975;292:771-4.
Knodell RG, Ishak G, Black C, Chen TS, Craig R, Kaplowitz N, et al. Formulation and application of numerical scoring system for activity in asymptomatic chronic active hepatitis. *Hepatology* 1981;1:431-5.

5 Other causes of parenchymal liver disease

S D Ryder, I J Beckingham

Autoimmune hepatitis

Autoimmune hepatitis is a relatively uncommon disease that mainly affects young women. The usual presentation is with fatigue, pain in the right upper quadrant of the abdomen, and polymyalgia or arthralgia associated with abnormal results of liver function tests. Other autoimmune diseases are present in 17% of patients with classic autoimmune hepatitis, predominantly thyroid disease, rheumatoid arthritis, and ulcerative colitis.

Autoimmune hepatitis is an important diagnosis as immunosuppressive drugs (prednisolone and azathioprine) produce lasting remission and an excellent prognosis. Although the condition can produce transient jaundice that seems to resolve totally, the process can continue at a subclinical level producing cirrhosis and irreversible liver failure. The diagnosis is based on detection of autoantibodies (antinuclear antibodies (60% positive), antismooth muscle antibodies (70%)) and high titres of immunoglobulins (present in almost all patients, usually IgG).

Metabolic causes of liver disease

Metabolic liver disease rarely presents as jaundice, and when it does the patient probably has end stage chronic liver disease.

Haemochromatosis

Haemochromatosis is the commonest inherited liver disease in the United Kingdom. It affects about 1 in 200 of the population and is 10 times more common than cystic fibrosis.

Haemochromatosis produces iron overload, and patients usually present with cirrhosis or diabetes due to excessive iron deposits in the liver or pancreas. The genetic defect responsible is a single base change at a locus of the HFE gene on chromosome 6, with this defect responsible for over 90% of cases in the United Kingdom. Genetic analysis is now available both for confirming the diagnosis and screening family members. The disease typically affects middle aged men. Menstruation and pregnancy probably account for the lower presentation in women.

Patients who are homozygous for the mutation should have regular venesection to prevent further tissue damage. Heterozygotes are asymptomatic and do not require treatment. Cardiac function is often improved by venesection but diabetes, arthritis, and hepatic fibrosis do not improve. This emphasises the need for early recognition and treatment.

Wilson's disease

Wilson's disease is a rare autosomal recessive cause of liver disease due to excessive deposition of copper within hepatocytes. Abnormal copper deposition also occurs in the basal ganglia and eyes. The defect lies in a decrease in production of the copper carrying enzyme ferroxidase. Unlike most other causes of liver disease, it is treatable and the prognosis is excellent provided that it is diagnosed before irreversible damage has occurred.

Patients may have a family history of liver or neurological disease and a greenish-brown corneal deposit of copper (a Kayser-Fleischer ring), which is often discernible only with a slit lamp. Most patients have a low caeruloplasmin level and low

> **About 40% of patients with autoimmune hepatitis present acutely with jaundice**

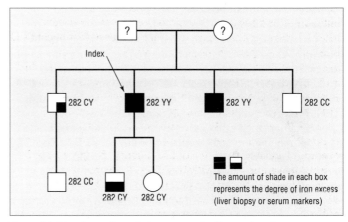

Figure 5.1 Use of genetic analysis to screen family members for haemochromatosis. The index case was a 45 year old man who presented with cirrhosis. His brothers were asymptomatic and had no clinical abnormalities. However, the brother who had inherited two abnormal genes (282YY) was found to have extensive iron loading on liver biopsy

---

Box 5.1 Presenting conditions in haemochromatosis

- Cirrhosis (70%)
- Diabetes (adult onset) (55%)
- Cardiac failure (20%)
- Arthropathy (45%)
- Skin pigmentation (80%)
- Sexual dysfunction (50%)

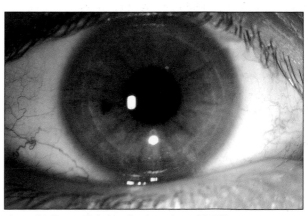

Figure 5.2 Kayser-Fleischer ring in patient with Wilson's disease

serum copper and high urinary copper concentrations. Liver biopsy confirms excessive deposition of copper.

Treatment is with penicillamine, which binds copper and increases urinary excretion. Patients who are unable to tolerate penicillamine are treated with trientene and oral zinc acetate. Asymptomatic siblings should be screened and treated in the same way.

Drug related hepatitis

Most drugs can cause liver injury. It is relatively uncommon for drug reactions to present as acute jaundice, and only 2-7% of hospital admissions for non-obstructive jaundice are drug related. Different drugs cause liver injury by a variety of mechanisms and with differing clinical patterns. In general terms, drug related jaundice can be due to predictable direct hepatotoxicity, such as is seen in paracetamol overdose, or idiosyncratic drug reactions.

Paracetamol poisoning
Paracetamol is usually metabolised by a saturable enzyme pathway. When the drug is taken in overdose, another metabolic system is used that produces a toxic metabolite that causes acute liver injury. Hepatotoxicity is common in paracetamol overdose, and prompt recognition and treatment is required. The lowest recorded fatal dose of paracetamol is 11 g, but genetic factors mean that most people would have to take considerably higher doses to develop fulminant liver failure.

Overdose with paracetamol is treated by acetylcysteine, which provides glutathione for detoxification of the toxic metabolites of paracetamol. This is generally a preventive measure, and decision to treat is based on the serum concentrations of paracetamol. It is important to be certain of the time that paracetamol was taken in order to interpret the treatment nomogram accurately. If there is doubt over the timing of ingestion treatment should be given.

Paracetamol poisoning is by far the commonest cause of fulminant liver failure in the United Kingdom and is an accepted indication for liver transplantation. As this is an acute liver injury, patients who survive without the need for transplantation will always regain normal liver function.

Idiosyncratic drug reactions
The idiosyncratic drug reactions are by their nature unpredictable. They can occur at any time during treatment and may still have an effect over a year after stopping the drug. The management of acute drug reactions is primarily stopping the potential causative agent, and if possible all drugs should be withheld until the diagnosis is definite. Idiosyncratic drug reactions can be severe, and they are an important cause of fulminant liver failure, accounting for between 15% and 20% of such cases. Any patient presenting with a severe drug reaction will require careful monitoring as recovery can be considerably delayed, particularly with drugs such as amiodarone, which has a long half life in blood.

The drug history must also include non-prescribed medications. Fulminant liver failure is well described in patients who have taken Chinese herbal medicine.

Cholestatic non-obstructive jaundice

Initial investigation of patients with jaundice and a cholestatic pattern on liver function tests is by ultrasonography. This will detect dilatation of the bile duct in most cases of extrahepatic biliary obstruction caused by tumour or stones and will also detect most metastatic liver tumours, the other main cause of

> **Wilson's disease should be suspected in any patient presenting with chronic hepatitis or cirrhosis under the age of 35**

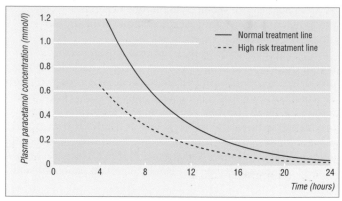

Figure 5.3 Thresholds for treatment of paracetamol poisoning in normal and high risk patients. Adapted from *British National Formulary*

Box 5.2 Common drugs producing hepatic idiosyncratic reactions

- Sodium valproate
- Non-steroidal anti-inflammatory drugs (diclofenac)
- Amiodarone
- Aspirin
- Methyldopa
- Isoniazid
- Minocycline

> **Complementary medicines may account for as much as 5% of all drug induced liver disease**

Box 5.3 Common drugs producing cholestatic reactions

- Chlorpromazine
- Oestrogens (hormone replacement therapy or contraceptive pill)
- Co-amoxiclav or flucloxacillin
- Chlorpropamide

cholestatic malignant jaundice. Dilatation of the biliary tree may not always be present in early biliary obstruction, and if doubt exists, either repeat ultrasonography or endoscopic retrograde cholangiopancreatography is advisable. Particular attention is required in patients with no apparent drug cause for their jaundice and in whom serological tests for other causes of cholestasis give negative results.

Primary biliary cirrhosis

Primary biliary cirrhosis is relatively common and mainly affects middle aged women. It typically presents as cholestatic jaundice, but with more widespread use of liver enzyme tests it is increasingly found at a presymptomatic stage because of raised alkaline phosphatase and γ-glutamyltransferase activities during investigation of associated symptoms such as pruritus. When patients present with jaundice, it is usually associated with cutaneous signs of chronic liver disease, xanthoma, and other extrahepatic features such as Sjögren's syndrome.

Primary biliary cirrhosis is immunologically mediated, and the presence of M2 antimitochondrial antibodies is diagnostic. Immunoglobulin titres, particularly IgM, are often raised. Liver biopsy is used to stage the disease rather than to confirm the diagnosis. Treatment with ursodeoxycholic acid has been shown to slow disease progression. Patients with advanced liver disease require liver transplantation.

Primary sclerosing cholangitis

Sclerosing cholangitis is characterised by progressive fibrosing inflammation of the bile ducts. The changes are often diffuse, but symptoms usually arise from dominant strictures at the hilum or within the extrahepatic bile ducts. Primary sclerosing cholangitis usually occurs in men younger than 50 years old and is associated with inflammatory bowel disease in 70-80% of cases. The incidence of primary sclerosing cholangitis in patients with ulcerative colitis is 2-10%. Cholangiocarcinoma develops in 20% to 30% of patients with primary sclerosing cholangitis and is an important cause of death in patients with ulcerative colitis.

Sclerosing cholangitis may be asymptomatic but usually presents with fluctuating jaundice, nausea, and pruritus. The diagnosis is suggested by cholangiography (endoscopic retrograde cholangiopancreatography, percutaneous transhepatic cholangiography, or magnetic resonance cholangiopancreatography). Multiple strictures with beading of ducts, duct pruning (scanty ducts), irregularities of the duct wall, and diverticula are typical features. Liver biopsy is a supplementary investigation that shows characteristic histological features in 30-40% of patients. Raised serum titres of smooth muscle antibody (70% of patients) and perinuclear antineutrophil cytoplasmic antibody (60%) may help diagnosis. Raised concentrations of serum CA19-9 tumour marker are highly suspicious of cholangiocarcinoma.

Treatment of primary sclerosing cholangitis is at present limited to the management of recurrent cholangitis. Treatment with ursodeoxycholic acid (7 mg/kg/day) may improve symptoms and liver function, but no strong evidence exists for its effectiveness. Dominant strictures may be improved with endoscopic dilatation or surgical resection. Liver transplantation is required for patients with deteriorating liver function with progressive secondary biliary cirrhosis.

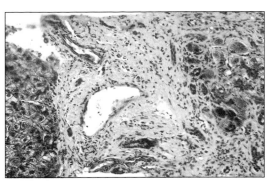

Figure 5.4 Broad fibrosis band in patient with primary biliary cirrhosis

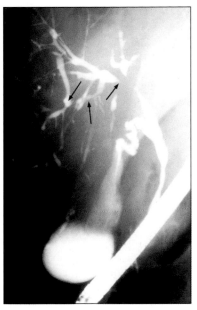

Figure 5.5 Endoscopic retrograde cholangiopancreatogram in patient with primary sclerosing cholangitis showing irregular stricturing and dilatation of intrahepatic bile ducts

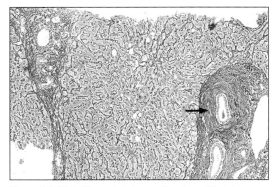

Figure 5.6 Liver biopsy specimen of patient with primary sclerosing cholangitis. Characteristic "onion skin" fibrosis is visible round portal tracts

Summary points

- Most drugs have potential to cause liver injury, and 2-7% of admissions with non-obstructive jaundice are for drug related hepatitis
- Herbal remedies and illegal drugs can also cause jaundice and liver damage
- Primary biliary cirrhosis typically presents as cholestatic jaundice in middle aged women
- Primary sclerosing cholangitis is associated with ulcerative colitis in 75% of cases, although the two may develop at different times
- Haemochromatosis is the commonest inherited liver disease in the United Kingdom, and a gene probe for clinical testing is now available

6 Portal hypertension—1: varices

J E J Krige, I J Beckingham

The portal vein carries about 1500 ml/min of blood from the small and large bowel, spleen, and stomach to the liver at a pressure of 5-10 mm Hg. Any obstruction or increased resistance to flow or, rarely, pathological increases in portal blood flow may lead to portal hypertension with portal pressures over 12 mm Hg. Although the differential diagnosis is extensive, alcoholic and viral cirrhosis are the leading causes of portal hypertension in Western countries, whereas liver disease due to schistosomiasis is the main cause in other areas of the world. Portal vein thrombosis is the commonest cause in children.

Increases in portal pressure cause development of a portosystemic collateral circulation with resultant compensatory portosystemic shunting and disturbed intrahepatic circulation. These factors are partly responsible for the important complications of chronic liver disease, including variceal bleeding, hepatic encephalopathy, ascites, hepatorenal syndrome, recurrent infection, and abnormalities in coagulation. Variceal bleeding is the most serious complication and is an important cause of death in patients with cirrhotic liver disease.

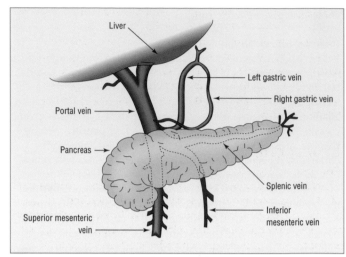

Figure 6.1 Anatomical relations of portal vein and branches

Varices

In Western countries variceal bleeding accounts for about 7% of episodes of gastrointestinal bleeding, although this varies according to the prevalence of alcohol related liver disease (11% in the United States, 5% in the United Kingdom). Patients with varices have a 30% lifetime risk of bleeding, and a third of those who bleed will die. Patients who have bled once from oesophageal varices have a 70% chance of bleeding again, and about a third of further bleeding episodes are fatal.

Several important considerations influence choice of treatment and prognosis. These include the natural course of the disease causing portal hypertension, location of the bleeding varices, residual hepatic function, presence of associated systemic disease, continuing drug or alcohol misuse, and response to specific treatment. The modified Child-Pugh classification identifies three risk categories that correlate well with survival.

Initial measures
Prompt resuscitation and restoration of circulating blood volume is vital and should precede any diagnostic studies. While their blood is being cross matched, patients should receive a rapid infusion of 5% dextrose and colloid solution until blood pressure is restored and urine output is adequate. Saline infusions may aggravate ascites and must be avoided. Patients who are haemodynamically unstable, elderly, or have concomitant cardiac or pulmonary disease should be monitored by using a pulmonary artery catheter as injudicious administration of crystalloids, combined with vasoactive drugs, can lead to the rapid onset of oedema, ascites, and hyponatraemia. Concentrations of clotting factors are often low, and fresh blood, fresh frozen plasma, and vitamin K_1 (phytomenadione) should be given. Platelet transfusions may be necessary. Sedatives should be avoided, although haloperidol is useful in patients with symptoms of alcohol withdrawal.

Box 6.1 Causes of portal hypertension

Increased resistance to flow

Prehepatic (portal vein obstruction)
- Congenital atresia or stenosis
- Thrombosis of portal vein
- Thrombosis of splenic vein
- Extrinsic compression (for example, tumours)

Hepatic
- Cirrhosis
- Acute alcoholic liver disease
- Congenital hepatic fibrosis
- Idiopathic portal hypertension (hepatoportal sclerosis)
- Schistosomiasis

Posthepatic
- Budd-Chiari syndrome
- Constrictive pericarditis

Increased portal blood flow
- Arterial-portal venous fistula
- Increased splenic flow

Table 6.1 Child-Pugh classification of liver failure

	No of points		
	1	**2**	**3**
Bilirubin (μmol/l)	<34	34-51	>51
Albumin (g/l)	>35	28-35	<28
Prothrombin time	<3	3-10	>10
Ascites	None	Slight	Moderate to severe
Encephalopathy	None	Slight	Moderate to severe

Grade A = 5-6 points, grade B = 7-9 points, grade C = 10-15 points.

Pharmacological control

Drug treatment, aimed at controlling the acute bleed and facilitating diagnostic endoscopy and emergency sclerotherapy, may be useful when variceal bleeding is rapid. Octreotide, a synthetic somatostatin analogue, reduces splanchnic blood flow when given intravenously as a constant infusion (50 µg/h) and can be used before endoscopy in patients with active bleeding. Vasopressin (0.4 units/min), or the long acting synthetic analogue terlipressin, combined with glyceryl trinitrate administered intravenously or transdermally through a skin patch is also effective but has more side effects than octreotide. Glyceryl trinitrate reduces the peripheral vasoconstriction caused by vasopressin and has an additive effect in lowering portal pressure.

Emergency endoscopy

Emergency diagnostic fibreoptic endoscopy is essential to confirm that oesophageal varices are present and are the source of bleeding. Most patients will have stopped bleeding spontaneously before endoscopy (60% of bleeds) or after drug treatment. Endotracheal intubation may be necessary during endoscopy, especially in patients who are bleeding heavily, encephalopathic, or unstable despite vigorous resuscitation. In 90% of patients variceal bleeding originates from oesophageal varices. These are treated by injection with sclerosant or by banding.

Sclerotherapy

In sclerotherapy a sclerosant solution (ethanolamine oleate or sodium tetradecyl sulphate) is injected into the bleeding varix or the overlying submucosa. Injection into the varix obliterates the lumen by thrombosis whereas injection into the submucosa produces inflammation followed by fibrosis. The first injection controls bleeding in 80% of cases. If bleeding recurs, the injection is repeated. Complications are related to toxicity of the sclerosant and include transient fever, dysphagia and chest pain, ulceration, stricture, and (rarely) perforation.

Band ligation

Band ligation is achieved by a banding device attached to the tip of the endoscope. The varix is aspirated into the banding chamber, and a trip wire dislodges a rubber band carried on the banding chamber, ligating the entrapped varix. One to three bands are applied to each varix, resulting in thrombosis. Band ligation eradicates oesophageal varices with fewer treatment sessions and complications than sclerotherapy.

Balloon tube tamponade

The balloon tube tamponade may be life saving in patients with active variceal bleeding if emergency sclerotherapy or banding is unavailable or not technically possible because visibility is obscured. In patients with active bleeding, an endotracheal tube should be inserted to protect the airway before attempting to place the oesophageal balloon tube.

The Minnesota balloon tube has four lumens, one for gastric aspiration, two to inflate the gastric and oesophageal balloons, and one above the oesophageal balloon for suction of secretions to prevent aspiration. The tube is inserted through the mouth, and correct siting within the stomach is checked by auscultation while injecting air through the gastric lumen. The gastric balloon is then inflated with 200 ml of air. Once fully inflated, the gastric balloon is pulled up against the oesophagogastric junction, compressing the submucosal varices. The tension is maintained by strapping a split tennis ball to the tube at the patient's mouth.

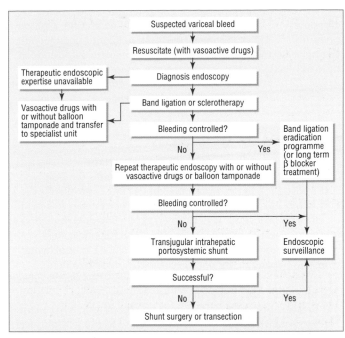

Figure 6.2 Algorithm for management of acute variceal haemorrhage

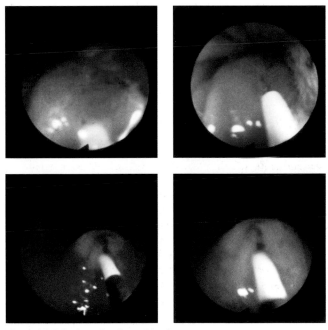

Figure 6.3 Injection of varices with sclerosant

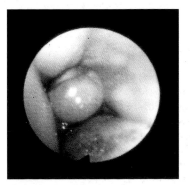

Figure 6.4 Band ligation of oesophageal varix

The oesophageal balloon is rarely required. The main complications are gastric and oesophageal ulceration, aspiration pneumonia, and oesophageal perforation. Continued bleeding during balloon tamponade indicates an incorrectly positioned tube or bleeding from another source. After resuscitation, and within 12 hours, the tube is removed and endoscopic treatment repeated.

Alternative management

Transjugular intrahepatic portosystemic shunt

Transjugular intrahepatic portosystemic shunt is the best procedure for patients whose bleeding is not controlled by endoscopy. It is effective only in portal hypertension of hepatic origin. The procedure is performed via the internal jugular vein under local anaesthesia with sedation. The hepatic vein is cannulated and a tract created through the liver parenchyma from the hepatic to the portal vein, with a needle under ultrasonographic and fluoroscopic guidance. The tract is dilated and an expandable metal stent inserted to create an intrahepatic portosystemic shunt. The success rate is excellent. Haemodynamic effects are similar to those found with surgical shunts, with a lower procedural morbidity and mortality.

Transjugular intrahepatic portosystemic shunting is an effective salvage procedure for stopping acute variceal haemorrhage, controlling bleeding from gastric varices, and congestive gastropathy after failure of medical and endoscopic treatment. However, because encephalopathy occurs in up to 25% of cases and up to 50% of shunts may occlude by one year, its primary role is to rescue failed endoscopy or as a bridge to subsequent liver transplantation.

Long term management

After the acute variceal haemorrhage has been controlled, treatment should be initiated to prevent rebleeding, which occurs in most patients.

Repeated endoscopic treatment

Repeated endoscopic treatment eradicates oesophageal varices in most patients, and provided that follow up is adequate serious recurrent variceal bleeding is uncommon. Because the underlying portal hypertension persists, patients remain at risk of developing recurrent varices and therefore require lifelong regular surveillance endoscopy.

Long term drug treatment

The use of β blockers after variceal bleeding has been shown to reduce portal blood pressures and lower the risk of further variceal bleeding. All patients should take β blockers unless they have contraindications. Best results are obtained when portal blood pressure is reduced by more than 20% of baseline or to below 12 mm Hg.

Surgical procedures

Patients with good liver function in whom endoscopic management fails or who live far from centres where endoscopic sclerotherapy services are available are candidates for surgical shunt procedures. A successful portosystemic shunt prevents recurrent variceal bleeding but is a major operation that may cause further impairment of liver function. Partial portacaval shunts with 8 mm interposition grafts are equally effective to other shunts in preventing rebleeding and have a low rate of encephalopathy.

Oesophageal transection and gastric devascularisation are now rarely performed but have a role in patients with portal

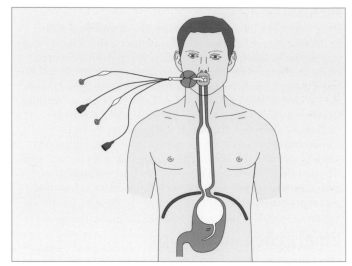

Figure 6.5 Minnesota balloon for tamponade of oesophageal varices

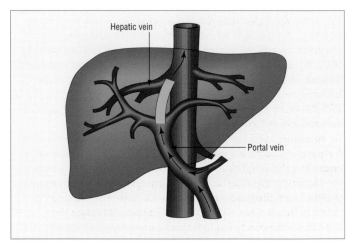

Figure 6.6 Transjugular intrahepatic portosystemic shunt

Box 6.2 Options for long term management
- Repeated endoscopic treatment
- Long term β blockers
- Surgical shunt
- Liver transplantation

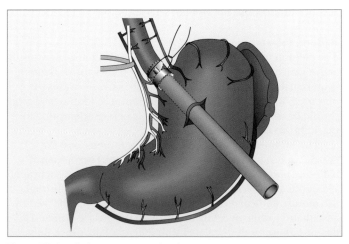

Figure 6.7 Surgical management of varices

and splenic vein thrombosis who are unsuitable for shunt procedures and continue to have serious variceal bleeding despite endoscopic and drug treatment.

Liver transplantation is the treatment of choice in advanced liver disease. Hepatic decompensation is the ultimate decompressive shunt for portal hypertension and also restores liver function. Transplantation treats other complications of portal hypertension and has one year and five year survival rates of 80% and 60% respectively.

Prophylactic management

Most patients with portal hypertension never bleed, and it is difficult to predict who will. Attempts at identifying patients at high risk of variceal haemorrhage by measuring the size or appearance of varices have been largely unsuccessful. β blockers have been shown to reduce the risk of bleeding, and all patients with varices should take them unless contraindicated.

Gastric varices and portal hypertensive gastropathy

Gastric varices are the source of bleeding in 5-10% of patients with variceal haemorrhage. Higher rates are reported in patients with left sided portal hypertension due to thrombosis of the splenic vein. Endoscopic control of gastric varices is difficult unless they are located on the proximal lesser curve in continuation with oesophageal varices. Endoscopic administration of cyanoacrylate monomer (superglue) is useful for gastric varices. The transjugular intrahepatic portosystemic shunt is increasingly used to control bleeding in this group.

Bleeding from portal hypertensive gastropathy accounts for 2-3% of bleeding episodes in cirrhosis. Although serious bleeding from these sources is uncommon, when it occurs its diffuse nature precludes the use of endoscopic treatment, and optimal management is with a combination of terlipressin and β blockers.

Further reading

Krige JEJ, Terblanche J. Endoscopic therapy in the management of oesophageal varices: injection sclerotherapy and variceal injection. In: Blumgart LH, ed. *Surgery of the liver and biliary tract.* London: Saunders, 2000:1885-1906

Sherlock S, Dooley J. Portal hypertension. In: *Diseases of the liver and biliary system.* Oxford: Blackwell Science, 1996

Sarin SK, Lamba GS, Kumar M, Misra A, Murthy NS. Comparison of endoscopic ligation and propranolol for the primary prevention of variceal bleeding. *N Engl J Med* 1999;340:988-93

Summary points

- Variceal bleeding is an important cause of death in cirrhotic patients
- Acute management consists of resuscitation and control of bleeding by sclerotherapy or balloon tamponade
- After a bleed patients require treatment to eradicate varices and lifelong surveillance to prevent further bleeds
- All patients with varices should take β blockers to reduce the risk of bleeding unless contraindicated by coexisting medical conditions
- Surgery is now rarely required for acute or chronic control of variceal bleeding

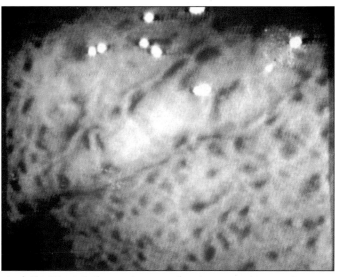

Figure 6.8 Hypertensive portal gastropathy

7   Portal hypertension–2. Ascites, encephalopathy, and other conditions

J E J Krige, I J Beckingham

Ascites

Ascites is caused by cirrhosis in 75% of cases, malignancy in 10%, and cardiac failure in 5%; other causes account for the remaining 10%. In most patients the history and examination will give valuable clues to the cause of the ascites—for example, signs of chronic liver disease, evidence of cardiac failure, or a pelvic mass. The formation of ascites in cirrhosis is due to a combination of abnormalities in both renal function and portal and splanchnic circulation. The main pathogenic factor is sodium retention. About half of patients with cirrhosis develop ascites during 10 years of observation. The development of ascites is an important event in chronic liver disease as half of cirrhotic patients with ascites die within two years.

Diagnosis

Ascites may not be clinically detectable when present in small volumes. In larger volumes, the classic findings of ascites are a distended abdomen with a fluid thrill or shifting dullness. Ascites must be differentiated from abdominal distension due to other causes such as obesity, pregnancy, gaseous distension of bowel, bladder distension, cysts, and tumours. Tense ascites may cause appreciable discomfort, difficulty in breathing, eversion of the umbilicus, herniae, and scrotal oedema. Rapid onset of ascites in patients with cirrhosis may be due to gastrointestinal haemorrhage, infection, portal venous thrombosis, or the development of a hepatocellular carcinoma. Ascites can also develop during a period of heavy alcohol misuse or excessive sodium intake in food or drugs. Ultrasonography is used to confirm the presence of minimal ascites and guide diagnostic paracentesis.

Successful treatment depends on an accurate diagnosis of the cause of ascites. Paracentesis with analysis of ascitic fluid is the most rapid and cost effective method of diagnosis. It should be done in patients with ascites of recent onset, cirrhotic patients with ascites admitted to hospital, or those with clinical deterioration. The most important analyses are quantitative cell counts, fluid culture, and calculation of the serum:ascites albumin gradient, which reflects differences in oncotic pressures and correlates with portal venous pressure. Patients with normal portal pressures have a serum:ascites albumin gradient less than 11 g/l, whereas patients with ascites associated with portal hypertension usually have a gradient above 11 g/l.

The traditional classification of transudative and exudative ascites based on ascitic fluid protein concentrations below and above 25 g/l is less useful than the serum:ascites albumin gradient because diuresis can affect the total ascitic protein concentration.

Treatment

The principal aim of treatment of symptomatic ascites in cirrhotic patients is to improve general comfort and quality of life. Most patients will respond to dietary sodium restriction and diuretic induced excretion of sodium and water, but other treatments are available for those who do not. Treatment does not necessarily improve the prognosis for patients with cirrhosis and may cause complications. Small amounts of ascites that are asymptomatic should not be treated.

Box 7.1 Causes of ascites

Portal hypertension
- Cirrhosis of liver
- Congestive heart failure
- Constrictive pericarditis
- Budd-Chiari syndrome
- Inferior vena cava obstruction

Hypoalbuminaemia
- Nephrotic syndrome
- Protein losing enteropathy

Neoplasms
- Peritoneal carcinomatosis
- Pseudomyxoma

Miscellaneous
- Pancreatic ascites
- Nephrogenic ascites (associated with maintenance haemodialysis)
- Myxoedema
- Meigs's syndrome

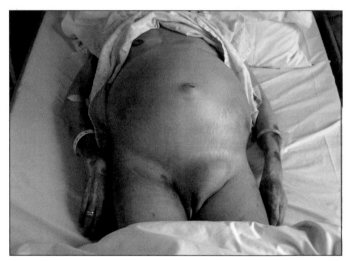

Figure 7.1 Tense ascites with umbilical and left inguinal hernias

---

Box 7.2 Analysis of ascitic fluid

- Evaluate macroscopic appearance (straw coloured, turbid, bloody, chylous)
- Cell count and differential
- Chemistry profile (protein, albumin, amylase)
- Cytology
- Gram stain and bacterial culture

Tests to consider ordering
- Adenosine deaminase (if tuberculosis is suspected)
- pH, lactate, lactate dehydrogenase (if bacterial peritonitis suspected)

Box 7.3 Classification of ascites by serum:ascites albumin gradient

High gradient (≥ 11 g/l)
- Cirrhosis
- Alcoholic hepatitis
- Cardiac ascites
- Fulminant hepatic failure
- Budd-Chiari syndrome
- Portal vein thrombosis
- Veno-occlusive disease

Low gradient (<11 g/l)
- Peritoneal carcinomatosis
- Tuberculous peritonitis
- Pancreatic ascites
- Biliary ascites
- Nephrotic syndrome
- Serositis of collagen, vascular disease

A crucial first step in treating ascites is to convince patients with alcoholic cirrhosis to abstain from alcohol. Abstinence for a few months can substantially improve the reversible component of alcoholic liver disease. Dietary salt restriction is the most important initial treatment. A low sodium diet of 1-1.5 g of salt (40-60 mmol/day) usually produces a net sodium loss, which may be sufficient in patients with mild ascites but is unpalatable and virtually impossible to adhere to in the long term. In practical terms a "no added salt" diet with levels of 80 mmol/day is the lowest that is generally sustainable. Fluid restriction is not needed for patients with cirrhotic ascites unless they have severe hyponatraemia (serum sodium < 120 mmol/l). Although conventional recommendations suggest bed rest, its value is not supported by controlled trials.

Most patients need dietary restrictions combined with diuretics. The usual diuretic regimen comprises single morning doses of oral spironolactone (an aldosterone antagonist), increasing the dose as necessary to a maximum of 400 mg/day. Dietary sodium restriction and dual diuretic therapy is effective in 90% of patients. The patient's weight, electrolyte concentrations, and renal function should be carefully monitored. Treatment should be cautious because of the dangers of iatrogenic complications from aggressive treatment. Patients with ascites and peripheral oedema may tolerate 1-2 kg loss per day, but loss of 0.5 kg should be the goal in patients without oedema. Potential complications during diuresis are encephalopathy, hypokalaemia, hyponatraemia, hypochloraemic alkalosis, and azotaemia.

Patients with tense ascites should have a total abdominal paracentesis, followed by a sodium restricted diet and oral diuretics. Options for patients who do not respond to routine medical treatment include serial therapeutic paracentesis, peritoneovenous shunt, transjugular intrahepatic portosystemic shunt, and liver transplantation. Serial therapeutic paracentesis should be performed as required, every two to three weeks. Albumin infusion is unnecessary if < 5 litres of fluid is removed.

Peritoneovenous shunts are seldom used because of problems with blockage and infection. They are reserved for patients who are resistant to diuretics, are not transplant candidates, and are unsuitable for paracentesis because of abdominal scars.

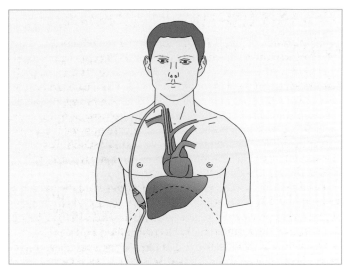

Figure 7.2 Denver peritoneovenous shunt

Box 7.4 Events precipitating hepatic encephalopathy in cirrhotic patients

Electrolyte imbalance
- Diuretics
- Vomiting
- Diarrhoea

Gastrointestinal bleeding
- Oesophageal and gastric varices
- Gastroduodenal erosions

Drugs
- Alcohol withdrawal
- Benzodiazepines

Infection
- Spontaneous bacterial peritonitis
- Urinary
- Chest

Constipation
- Dietary protein overload

Hepatic encephalopathy

Hepatic encephalopathy is a reversible state of impaired cognitive function or altered consciousness that occurs in patients with liver disease or portosystemic shunts. The typical features of hepatic encephalopathy include impaired consciousness (drowsiness), monotonous speech, flat affect, metabolic tremor, muscular incoordination, impaired handwriting, fetor hepaticus, upgoing plantar responses, hypoactive or hyperactive reflexes, and decerebrate posturing. Hepatic coma, especially in alcoholic patients, should be diagnosed only after coma due to intracranial space occupying and vascular lesions, trauma, infection, epilepsy, and metabolic, endocrine, and drug induced causes has been excluded. Hepatic encephalopathy is a hallmark of deteriorating liver function, and patients should be assessed early for liver transplantation.

Hepatocellular insufficiency and portosystemic shunting may act separately or in combination to cause encephalopathy. Almost all cases of clinically apparent hepatic encephalopathy occur in patients with cirrhosis. Less than 5% occur in patients with non-cirrhotic forms of portal hypertension. However, a disproportionately large proportion of patients with surgical and radiological portosystemic shunts develop severe, often intractable, hepatic encephalopathy. A combination of impaired

---

Box 7.5 Drugs that can cause hepatic encephalopathy

- Barbiturates
- Analgesics
- Other sedatives

Box 7.6 Treatment of hepatic encephalopathy

- Identify the precipitating factors
- Stop diuretics
- Check serum Na$^+$, K$^+$, and urea concentration
- Empty bowels of nitrogen containing content
    Control bleeding
    Protein-free diet
- Lactulose
- Neomycin (1 g four times a day by mouth for 1 week)
- Maintain energy, fluid, and electrolyte balance
- Increase dietary protein slowly with recovery

hepatic and renal function is often associated with hepatic encephalopathy. About half these patients have diuretic induced renal impairment and half have functional renal failure.

Drugs are implicated in one quarter of patients with hepatic encephalopathy. Another quarter of cases are precipitated by haemorrhage in the gastrointestinal tract. This is often associated with deep and prolonged coma. The combination of gastrointestinal haemorrhage and hepatic encephalopathy indicates a poor prognosis. A small proportion of cases are precipitated by excess dietary protein, hypokalaemic alkalosis, constipation, and deterioration of liver function secondary to drugs, toxins, viruses, or hepatocellular carcinoma.

The treatment of hepatic encephalopathy is empirical and relies largely on establishing the correct diagnosis, identifying and treating precipitating factors, emptying the bowels of blood, protein, and stool, attending to electrolyte and acid-base imbalance, and the selective use of benzodiazepine antagonists. Non-absorbable disaccharides, such as lactulose or lactitol, are the mainstay of treatment. Antibiotics and protein restriction (40 g/day) can be used if there is no response. In intractable cases, closure of surgical shunts should be considered.

Hepatorenal syndrome

Hepatorenal syndrome is an acute oliguric renal failure resulting from intense intrarenal vasoconstriction in otherwise normal kidneys. It occurs in patients with chronic liver disease (usually cirrhosis, portal hypertension, or ascites) or acute liver failure; a clinical cause is often not found, treatment is often ineffective, and prognosis is poor. Hepatorenal syndrome is prevented by avoiding excessive diuresis and by early recognition of electrolyte imbalance, bleeding, or infection. Potentially nephrotoxic drugs such as aminoglycosides and non-steroidal anti-inflammatories should be avoided.

Patients with hepatorenal syndrome should have blood cultures taken and any bacteraemia treated. Most patients with liver disease who develop azotaemia will have prerenal failure or acute tubular necrosis. The diagnosis of hepatorenal syndrome is one of exclusion, and it should not be diagnosed until all potentially reversible causes of renal failure have been excluded. The common potentially reversible causes are sepsis, excessive diuresis or paracentesis, and nephrotoxic drugs. All patients suspected to have hepatorenal syndrome should be given an intravenous colloid infusion to exclude intravascular hypovolaemia as a cause of prerenal azotaemia. Liver transplantation, if otherwise appropriate and feasible, is the only truly effective treatment, and patients have a poor prognosis.

Spontaneous bacterial peritonitis

Spontaneous bacterial peritonitis is usually the consequence of bacteraemia due to defects in the hepatic reticuloendothelial system and in the peripheral destruction of bacteria by neutrophils. This allows secondary seeding of bacteria in the ascitic fluid, which is deficient in antibacterial activity.

Clinical signs may be minimal, and a diagnostic paracentesis should be performed in any cirrhotic patient who suddenly deteriorates or presents with fever or abdominal pain. A polymorphonuclear neutrophil count $>500 \times 10^6/l$ is indicative of spontaneous bacterial peritonitis. Treatment with intravenous broad spectrum antibiotics should be started while awaiting the results of culture of ascitic fluid. Although the mortality associated with acute spontaneous bacterial peritonitis decreases with early treatment, it is still high (about 50%) and is related to the severity of the underlying liver disease.

In patients with cirrhosis and ascites spontaneous bacterial peritonitis is a common cause of sudden deterioration and may be present without any abdominal symptoms or signs

---

Box 7.7 Characteristic findings associated with hepatorenal syndrome

- Ascites (but not necessarily jaundice) is usually present
- Hyponatraemia is usual
- Hepatic encephalopathy is commonly present
- Blood pressure is reduced compared with previous pressures recorded in patient
- Pronounced oliguria
- Low renal sodium concentration (<10mmol/l)
- Urinary protein and casts are minimal or absent

Summary points

- Cirrhosis is the commonest cause of ascites (90%)
- Ninety per cent of cases can be managed by sodium restriction and diuretics
- Hepatic encephalopathy is most commonly precipitated by drugs or gastrointestinal haemorrhage
- Non-steroidal anti-inflammatory drugs should be avoided in cirrhotic patients as they can cause renal failure

---

Further reading

Sherlock S, Dooley J. Diseases of the liver and biliary system. Oxford: Blackwell Scientific, 1996

Riordan SM, Williams R. Management of liver failure. In: Blumgart LH, ed. *Surgery of the liver and biliary tract*. London: W B Saunders, 2000:1825-38

Box 7.8 Spontaneous bacterial peritonitis

- An infection of ascites that occurs in the absence of a local infectious source
- Mainly a complication of cirrhotic ascites
- Prevalence is 15% to 20% (including culture negative cases)
- Caused by Gram negative enteric bacteria in >70% of cases

8 Liver tumours

I J Beckingham, J E J Krige

Tumours of the liver may be cystic or solid, benign or malignant. Most are asymptomatic, with patients having normal liver function, and they are increasingly discovered incidentally during ultrasonography or computed tomography. Although most tumours are benign and require no treatment, it is important for non-specialists to be able to identify lesions that require further investigation and thus avoid unnecessary biopsy. Modern imaging combined with recent technical advances in liver surgery can now offer many patients safe and potentially curative resections for malignant, as well as benign, conditions affecting the liver.

Cystic liver lesions

Cystic lesions of the liver are easily identified by ultrasonography. Over 95% are simple cysts. Asymptomatic cysts are regarded as congenital malformations and require no further investigation or treatment as complications are rare. Aspiration and injection of sclerosants should be avoided as it may cause bleeding and infection and does not resolve the cyst. Rarely, simple cysts can grow very large and produce compressive symptoms. These are managed by limited surgical excision of the cyst wall (cyst fenestration), which can usually be done laparoscopically.

About half of patients with simple cysts have two or more cysts. True polycystic liver disease is seen as part of adult polycystic kidney disease, an uncommon autosomal dominant disease that progresses to renal failure. Patients nearly always have multiple renal cysts, which usually precede development of liver cysts. Liver function is normal, and most patients have no symptoms. Occasionally the cysts cause pain because of distension of the liver capsule, and such patients may require cyst fenestration or partial liver resection.

Thick walled cysts and those containing septa, nodules, or echogenic fluid may be cystic tumours (cystadenoma, cystadenocarcinoma) or infective cysts (hydatid cysts and abscesses; see later article in this series), and patients should be referred for specialist surgical opinion. Cystic dilatations of the bile ducts (Caroli's disease) are important as they may produce cholangitis and are premalignant with the potential to develop into cholangiocarcinoma.

Benign tumours

Benign liver tumours are common and are usually asymptomatic. Although most need no treatment, it is important to be able to differentiate them from malignant lesions.

Haemangiomas
Haemangiomas are the commonest benign solid tumours of the liver, with an incidence in the general population of around 3%. Those over 10 cm in diameter occasionally produce non-specific symptoms of abdominal discomfort and fullness and, rarely, fever, thrombocytopenia, and hypofibrinogenaemia due to thrombosis in the cavernous cavities. Malignant transformation and spontaneous rupture are rare. Contrast enhanced computed tomography is usually sufficient to diagnose most haemangiomas, and in equivocal cases magnetic

> Liver biopsy of a tumour mass should be reserved for patients with suspected malignancy who are not suitable for surgery and in whom the diagnosis may have clinical impact—for example, ovarian or neuroendocrine tumours, carcinoid, or lymphoma

Box 8.1 Characteristics of simple cysts
- Thin walled
- Contain clear fluid
- Contain no septa or debris
- Surrounded by normal liver tissue
- Usually asymptomatic
- Present in 1% of population

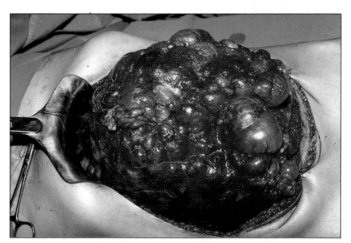

Figure 8.1 Polycystic liver disease

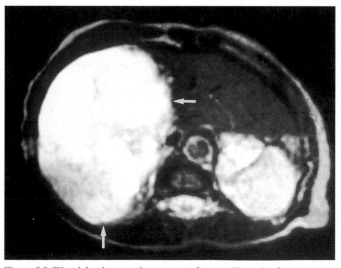

Figure 8.2 T2 weighted magnetic resonance image of large benign haemangioma showing light bulb sign

resonance imaging or technetium-99 labelled red blood cell scintigraphy will confirm the diagnosis. Angiography and biopsy are seldom required. Resection is indicated only for large symptomatic tumours.

Liver cell adenoma and focal nodular hyperplasia

These uncommon tumours occur predominantly in women of childbearing age. Liver cell adenoma became more prevalent with the widespread use of oral contraceptives in the 1960s, but the reduced oestrogen content of modern contraceptives has made it less common. Most patients present with pain due to rapid tumour growth, intratumour haemorrhage, or the sensation of a mass. The risk of rupture is 10%, and malignant transformation is found in 10% of resected specimens. Patients should have liver resection to prevent these events.

Focal nodular hyperplasia is not related to use of oral contraceptives, is usually asymptomatic, and is not premalignant. Mass lesions usually contain a central stellate scar on computed tomography and magnetic resonance imaging. It does not require treatment unless symptomatic.

In a small proportion of patients a firm radiological diagnosis cannot be reached and the distinction from a malignant liver tumour is uncertain. Histological distinction between focal nodular hyperplasia and cirrhosis and between liver cell adenoma and well differentiated hepatocellular carcinoma can be difficult with tru-cut biopsy or fine needle aspiration samples, and biopsy has the added risk of bleeding and tumour seeding. The histology should therefore be determined by surgical resection, which in specialist centres has a mortality of < 1%.

Malignant tumours

Hepatocellular carcinoma

Hepatocellular carcinoma is uncommon in the United Kingdom and accounts for only 2% of all cancers. Worldwide there are over one million new cases a year, with an annual incidence of 100 per 100 000 men in parts of South Africa and South East Asia. The incidence of hepatocellular carcinoma is increased in areas with high carrier rates of hepatitis B and C and in patients with haemochromatosis. More than 80% of hepatocellular carcinomas occur in patients with cirrhotic livers. Once viral infection is established it takes about 10 years for patients to develop chronic hepatitis, 20 years to develop cirrhosis, and 30 years to develop carcinoma. In African and Asian countries aflatoxin, produced as a result of contamination of imperfectly stored staple crops by *Aspergillus flavus*, seems to be an independent risk factor for the development of hepatocellular carcinoma, probably through mutation of the p53 suppressor gene. Seasonal variation in incidence is seen in these countries.

In patients with cirrhosis, the diagnosis should be suspected when there is deterioration in liver function, an acute complication (ascites, encephalopathy, variceal bleed, jaundice), or development of upper abdominal pain and fever. Ultrasonography will identify most tumours, and the presence of a discrete mass within a cirrhotic liver, together with an α fetoprotein concentration above 500 ng/ml is diagnostic. Biopsy is unnecessary and should be avoided to reduce the risk of tumour seeding. Surgical resection is the only treatment that can offer cure. However, owing to local spread of tumour and severity of pre-existing cirrhosis, such treatment is feasible in less than 20% of patients. Average operative mortality is 12% in cirrhotic patients, and five year survival is around 15%.

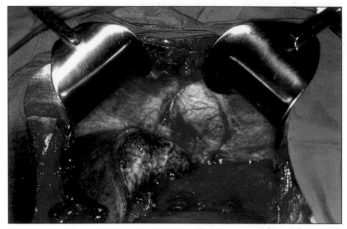

Figure 8.3 Intraoperative view after left hepatectomy—raw surfaces of liver are coated with fibrin glue after resection to aid haemostasis and prevent small bile leaks

> **Hepatocellular carcinoma is the commonest malignant tumour worldwide**

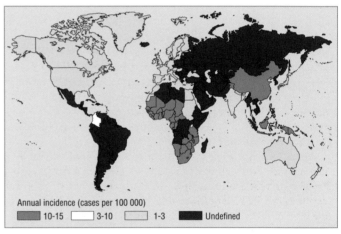

Annual incidence (cases per 100 000)
■ 10-15   □ 3-10   □ 1-3   ■ Undefined

Figure 8.4 Distribution of hepatocellular carcinoma

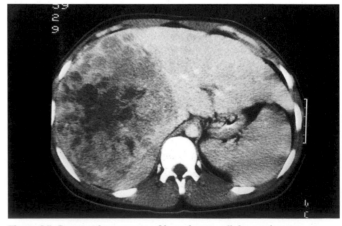

Figure 8.5 Computed tomogram of large hepatocellular carcinoma

Patients with cirrhosis and small (<5 cm) tumours should have liver transplantation. Injection of alcohol or radiofrequency ablation can improve survival in patients with small tumours who are unsuitable for transplantation. For larger tumours, transarterial embolisation with lipiodol and cytotoxic drugs (cisplatin or doxorubicin) may induce tumour necrosis in some patients.

In patients without cirrhosis, hepatocellular carcinomas usually present late with an abdominal mass and abnormal liver function. Computed tomography has a greater sensitivity and specificity than ultrasonography, particularly for tumours smaller than 1 cm. α Fetoprotein concentrations are raised in 80% of patients but may also be raised in patients with testicular or germ cell tumours.

Fibrolamellar carcinoma is an important subtype of hepatocellular carcinoma. It occurs in patients without cirrhosis or previous hepatitis infection. It accounts for 15% of hepatocellular carcinoma in the Western hemisphere. The prognosis is better than for other hepatocellular carcinomas, with a five year survival of 40-50% after resection.

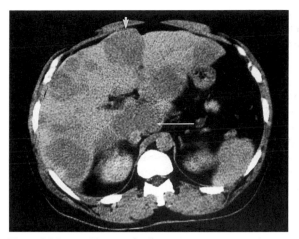
Figure 8.6 Inoperable extensive liver metastases

Metastatic tumours

Liver metastases are common and are found in 40% of all patients dying from cancer. They are most frequently associated with carcinomas of the gastrointestinal tract (colorectal, pancreas, and stomach) but are nearly as common in carcinomas of the bronchus, breast, ovary, and lymphoma. With the exception of liver metastases of colorectal cancer, tumour deposits are almost always multiple and seldom amenable to resection.

Colorectal liver metastases

Around 8-10 % of patients undergoing curative resection of colorectal tumours have isolated liver metastases suitable for liver resection, equivalent to around 1000 patients in the United Kingdom a year. Half will have metastases at the time of diagnosis of the primary tumour (synchronous metastases) and most of the rest will develop metastases within the next three years (metachronous metastases).

Without surgical resection the five year survival rate for all patients with liver metastases is zero, compared with an overall five year survival after resection of 30%. Patients most suited for resection are those with fewer than three or four metastases in one lobe of the liver, but tumours need not be confined to one lobe. The principle of complete tumour removal, however, remains a prerequisite, and one limitation is the need to leave enough liver to function. This depends both on the extent and distribution of the tumour burden and the general fitness of the patient and his or her liver. The liver has an enormous capacity for regeneration. A fit patient with a healthy liver will regenerate a 75% resection within three months. Age is only a relative contraindication, and several series have reported low mortality in septuagenarians.

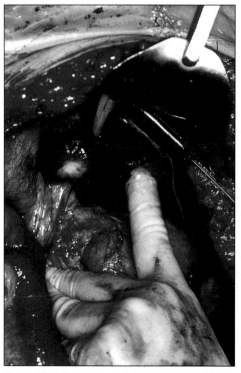
Figure 8.7 Solitary metastasis in segment IV of liver

Liver resection

Liver resection has advanced rapidly over the past two decades because of several important developments. The segmental anatomy of the liver, with each of the eight segments supplied by its own branch of the hepatic artery, portal vein, and bile duct, was first described by Couinaud in 1957. It is now possible to remove each of these segments individually when required, reducing the amount of normal liver unnecessarily removed.

Subsequently surgical techniques have been developed to divide the liver parenchyma, either by crushing with a clamp or

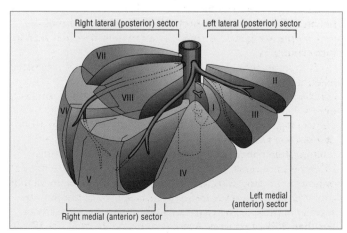
Figure 8.8 Couinaud's segmental anatomy of liver

by ultrasonic dissection, allowing the vascular and biliary radicals to be individually ligated. Blood loss has been reduced by occlusion of the vascular inflow (Pringle manoeuvre) and where possible the appropriate hepatic vein, together with lowering of the central venous pressure during resection, and blood transfusion is now unnecessary in 60% of major liver resections.

Improvements have also occurred in anaesthetic and postoperative care, including epidural anaesthesia to reduce postoperative pain and chest complications and the ability to manage postoperative fluid or bile collections by radiological or endoscopic drainage. These developments mean that the median hospital stay for patients having liver resection is now 7-10 days and mortality is around 5%. Liver resection has evolved from a hazardous bloody procedure into a routine operation.

Summary points

- Simple liver cysts are common, benign, and require no treatment
- Patients with solitary liver masses should be referred to a hepatobiliary surgeon and liver biopsy avoided
- Liver resection is a safe procedure in non-cirrhotic patients, with a mortality around 5%
- 10% of patients with colorectal cancer develop potentially curable liver metastases and should have six monthly liver ultrasonography or computed tomography
- Five year survival after resection of colorectal metastases is >30%

Further reading

- Blumgart LH, Jarnogin W, Fang Y. Liver resection. In: Blumgart LH, ed. *Surgery of the liver and biliary tract.* London: WB Saunders, 2000:1639-1714
- Launois B, Jamieson GG. *Modern operative techniques in liver surgery.* Edinburgh: Churchill Livingstone, 1993
- Neeleman N, Andersson R. Repeated liver resection for recurrent liver cancer. *Br J Surg* 1996;83:885-92

9 Liver abscesses and hydatid disease

J E J Krige, I J Beckingham

Liver abscesses are caused by bacterial, parasitic, or fungal infection. Pyogenic abscesses account for three quarters of hepatic abscess in developed countries. Elsewhere, amoebic abscesses are more common, and, worldwide, amoebae are the commonest cause.

Pyogenic liver abscesses

Aetiology
Most pyogenic liver abscesses are secondary to infection originating in the abdomen. Cholangitis due to stones or strictures is the commonest cause, followed by abdominal infection due to diverticulitis or appendicitis. In 15% of cases no cause can be found (cryptogenic abscesses). Compromised host defences have been implicated in the development of cryptogenic abscess and may have a role in the aetiology of most hepatic abscesses. Diabetes mellitus has been noted in 15% of adults with liver abscesses.

Microbiology
Most patients presenting with pyogenic liver abscesses have a polymicrobial infection usually with Gram negative aerobic and anaerobic organisms. Most organisms are of bowel origin, with *Escherichia coli, Klebsiella pneumoniae,* bacteroides, enterococci, anaerobic streptococci, and microaerophilic streptococci being most common. Staphylococci, haemolytic streptococci, and *Streptococcus milleri* are usually present if the primary infection is bacterial endocarditis or dental sepsis. Immunosuppression due to AIDS, intensive chemotherapy, and transplantation has increased the number of abscesses due to fungal or opportunistic organisms.

Clinical features
The classic presentation is with abdominal pain, swinging fever, and nocturnal sweating, vomiting, anorexia, malaise, and weight loss. The onset may be insidious or occult in elderly people, and patients may present with a primary infection (such as diverticulitis or appendicitis) before developing symptoms from their liver abscess. Single abscesses tend to be gradual in onset and are often cryptogenic. Multiple abscesses are associated with more acute systemic features and the cause is more often identified.

Clinically, the liver is enlarged and tender, and percussion over the lower ribs aggravates the pain. Clinical jaundice occurs only in the late stage unless there is suppurative cholangitis. Some patients do not have right upper quadrant pain or hepatomegaly and present with fever of unknown origin.

Laboratory investigations
Two thirds of patients have appreciable leucocytosis, often accompanied by anaemia of chronic infection and a raised erythrocyte sedimentation rate. The alkaline phosphatase activity is generally raised, hypoalbuminaemia is present, and serum transaminase activity may be marginally abnormal.

Plain abdominal radiography may show hepatomegaly, sometimes with an air fluid level in the abscess cavity. The right diaphragm is often raised, with a pleural reaction or pneumonic consolidation. Ultrasonography is the preferred initial method of imaging as it is non-invasive, cost effective, and can be used to

---

Box 9.1 Typical features of pyogenic liver abscess

- Right upper quadrant pain and tenderness
- Nocturnal fevers and sweats
- Anorexia and weight loss
- Raised right hemidiaphragm in chest radiograph
- Raised white cell count and erythrocyte sedimentation rate with mild anaemia

---

Box 9.2 Origins and causes of pyogenic liver abscess

- Biliary tract
  Gall stones
  Cholangiocarcinoma
  Strictures
- Portal vein
  Appendicitis
  Diverticulitis
  Crohn's disease
- Hepatic artery
  Dental infection
  Bacterial endocarditis

- Direct extension of:
  Gall bladder empyema
  Perforated peptic ulcer
  Subphrenic abscess
- Trauma
- Iatrogenic
  Liver biopsy
  Blocked biliary stent
- Cryptogenic
- Secondary infection of liver cyst

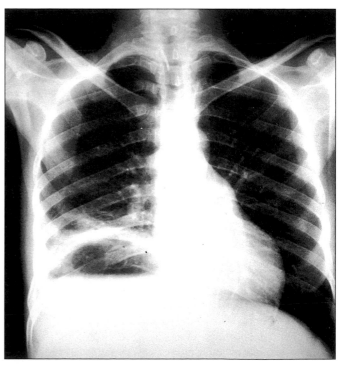

Figure 9.1 Chest radiograph showing air-fluid level and raised right hemidiaphragm in pyogenic liver abscess

guide aspiration to identify the causative organism. Computed tomography is useful to identify other intra-abdominal abscesses. Endoscopic retrograde cholangiopancreatography is used to define the site and cause of biliary obstruction and to allow biliary stenting and drainage.

Treatment

Empirical broad spectrum parenteral antibiotic treatment should be started as soon as an abscess is diagnosed. Antibiotics should include penicillin, an aminoglycoside, and metronidazole, which are effective against *E coli, K pneumoniae,* bacteroides, enterococcus, and anaerobic streptococci. In elderly people and those with impaired renal function a third generation cephalosporin should be used instead of an aminoglycoside. The regimen should be modified after culture has identified the infective organism. Treatment is continued for two to four weeks depending on the number of abscesses, the clinical response, and the potential toxicity of the chosen regimen.

Antibiotics alone are effective in only a few patients, and most patients will require percutaneous aspiration or catheter drainage guided by ultrasonography or computed tomography. In all cases the underlying cause should be sought and treated.

Early diagnosis, treatment with appropriate antibiotics, and selective drainage have substantially reduced mortality. Factors that increase the risk of death include shock, adult respiratory distress syndrome, disseminated intravascular coagulation, immunodeficiency states, severe hypoalbuminaemia, diabetes, ineffective surgical drainage, and associated malignancy.

Amoebic liver abscess

About 10% of the world's population is chronically infected with *Entamoeba histolytica.* Amoebiasis is the third commonest parasitic cause of death, surpassed only by malaria and schistosomiasis. The prevalence of infection varies widely, and it occurs most commonly in tropical and subtropical climates. Overcrowding and poor sanitation are the main predisposing factors.

Pathogenesis
The parasite is transmitted through the faeco-oral route with the ingestion of viable protozoal cysts. The cyst wall disintegrates in the small intestine, releasing motile trophozoites. These migrate to the large bowel, where pathogenic strains may cause invasive disease. Mucosal invasion results in the formation of flask-shaped ulcers through which amoebae gain access to the portal venous system. The abscess is usually solitary and affects the right lobe in 80% of cases. The abscess contains sterile pus and reddish-brown ("anchovy paste") liquefied necrotic liver tissue. Amoebae are occasionally present at the periphery of the abscess.

Clinical presentation and diagnosis
Patients may have had symptoms from a few days to several weeks before presentation. Pain is a prominent feature, and the patient appears toxic, febrile, and chronically ill.

The diagnosis is based on clinical, serological, and radiological features. The patient is usually resident in an endemic area or has visited one recently, although there may be no history of diarrhoea. Patients commonly have leucocytosis with 70-80% polymorphs (eosinophilia is not a feature), a raised erythrocyte sedimentation rate, and moderate anaemia In patients with severe disease and multiple abscesses, alkaline phosphatase activity and bilirubin concentration are raised. Stools may contain cysts, or in the case of dysentery, haematophagous trophozoites.

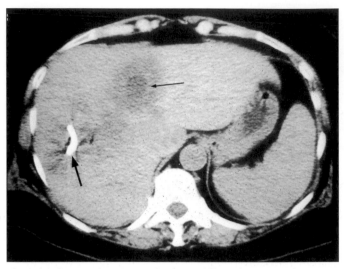

Figure 9.2 Computed tomogram showing multifocal liver abscess in segment IV. Note drain and second abscess in segments VII and VIII

Box 9.3 Drainage requirements for liver abscesses

- None—multiple small abscesses that respond to antibiotics (Obstruction of bile duct must be excluded as a cause and endoscopic retrograde cholangiopancreatography with stenting performed if necessary)
- Percutaneous aspiration—abscesses <6 cm
- Percutaneous catheter drainage—abscesses ≥6 cm
- Open surgery
  Failed percutaneous drainage
  Very large or multilocular abscesses
  Associated intra-abdominal infection requiring surgery such as bile duct stones

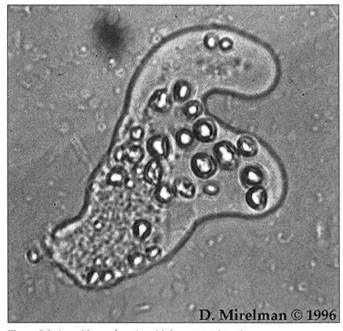

Figure 9.3 Amoebic trophozoite with large pseudopod

Box 9.4 Symptoms of amoebic liver abscess

- Pain
- Enlarged liver with maximal tenderness over abscess
- Intermittent fever (38-39°C)
- Night sweats
- Weight loss
- Nausea
- Vomiting
- Cough
- Dyspnoea

Chest radiography usually shows a raised right hemidiaphragm with atelectasis or pleural effusion. Ultrasonography shows the size and position of the abscess and is useful when aspiration is necessary and to assess response to treatment. Serological tests provide a rapid means of confirming the diagnosis, but the results may be misleading in endemic areas because of previous infection. Indirect haemagglutination titres for entamoeba are raised in over 90% of patients. In areas where amoebiasis is uncommon, failure to consider the infection may delay diagnosis.

Serious complications occur as a result of secondary infection or rupture into adjacent structures such as pleural, pericardial, or peritoneal spaces. Two thirds of ruptures occur intraperitoneally and one third intrathoracically.

Treatment

Ninety five per cent of uncomplicated amoebic abscesses resolve with metronidazole alone (800 mg, three times a day for five days). Supportive measures such as adequate nutrition and pain relief are important. Clinical symptoms usually improve greatly within 24 hours. Lower doses of metronidazole are often effective in invasive disease but may fail to eliminate the intraluminal infection, allowing clinical relapses to occur. After the amoebic abscess has been treated, patients are prescribed diloxanide furoate 500 mg, eight hourly for seven days, to eliminate intestinal amoebae.

Patients should have ultrasonographically guided needle aspiration if serology gives negative results or the abscess is large (> 10 cm), if they do not respond to treatment, or if there is impending peritoneal, pleural, or pericardial rupture. Surgical drainage is required only if the abscess has ruptured causing amoebic peritonitis or if the patient has not responded to drugs despite aspiration or catheter drainage.

Hydatid disease

Hydatid disease in humans is caused by the dog tapeworm, *Echinococcus granulosus*. Dogs are the definitive host. Ova are shed in the faeces and then infect the natural intermediate hosts such as sheep or cattle. Hydatid disease is endemic in many sheep raising countries. Increasing migration and world travel have made hydatidosis a global problem of increasing importance.

Human infection follows accidental ingestion of ova passed in dog faeces. The ova penetrate the intestinal wall and pass through the portal vein to the liver, lung, and other tissues. Hydatid cysts can develop anywhere in the body, but two thirds occur in the liver and one quarter in the lungs.

Presentation

Patients with a liver hydatid may present either with liver enlargement and right upper quadrant pain due to pressure from the cyst or acutely with a complication. Complications include rupture of the cyst into the peritoneal cavity, which results in urticaria, anaphylactic shock, eosinophilia, and implantation into the omentum and other viscera. Cysts may compress or erode into a bile duct causing pain, jaundice, or cholangitis, or the cyst may become infected secondary to a bile leak.

Diagnsosis and treatment

Ultrasonography and computed tomography will show the size, position, and number of liver cysts and any extrahepatic cysts. Around 10% of patients with a liver cyst will also have a lung hydatid on chest radiography. Eosinophilia is present in 40% of patients. The diagnosis is confirmed by haemagglutination and complement fixation tests. Endoscopic retrograde

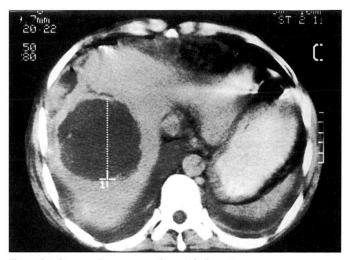

Figure 9.4 Computed tomogram of amoebic liver abscess

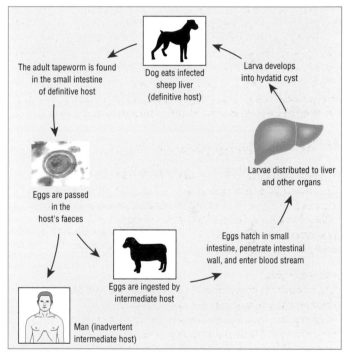

Figure 9.5 Lifecycle of *Echinococcus granulosus*

The adult tapeworm is found in the small intestine of definitive host

Dog eats infected sheep liver (definitive host)

Larva develops into hydatid cyst

Eggs are passed in the host's faeces

Larvae distributed to liver and other organs

Eggs hatch in small intestine, penetrate intestinal wall, and enter blood stream

Eggs are ingested by intermediate host

Man (inadvertent intermediate host)

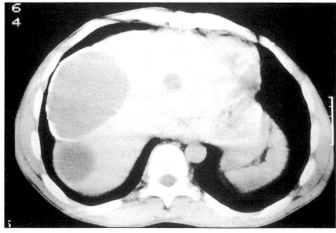

Figure 9.6 Hydatid cyst in right lobe of liver with calcifcation in the wall

cholangiopancreatography will show communication between the cyst and the bile ducts if patients are jaundiced, their serum alkaline phosphatase or γ-glutamyltransferase activity is raised, or their bilirubin concentration increased.

All symptomatic cysts require surgical removal to prevent complications. Small densely calcified cysts ("golf ball" appearance) signify death of the parasite and require no further treatment. Careful isolation of the operative field by abdominal swabs soaked in scolicidal fluid is essential to prevent spillage and formation of intraperitoneal cysts. The cyst fluid is aspirated and replaced by a scolicidal agent such as 0.5% sodium hypochlorite or 0.5% silver nitrate. Scolicidal solutions should not be injected if there is a bile leak because of possible chemical injury to the biliary epithelium.

After decompression, the cyst and contents are carefully shelled out by peeling the endocyst off the host ectocyst layer along its cleavage plane. The fibrous host wall of the residual cavity should be carefully examined for any bile leakage from biliary-cyst communications, which are then sutured. The cavity is drained and filled with omentum.

Conservative surgery is effective in most cysts, and liver resection is seldom necessary. Albendazole, flubendazole, or praziquantel are given for two weeks postoperatively to prevent recurrence. Drug treatment can be used in patients unfit for surgery and in those with disseminated, recurrent, or inoperable disease and as an adjuvant in complex surgery. These drugs must be used cautiously and patients monitored for side effects, which include depression of bone marrow activity and liver and renal toxicity.

Further reading

Krige JEJ. Pyogenic liver abscess. In: Kirsch R, Robson S, Trey C, eds. *Diagnosis and management of liver disease.* London: Chapman and Hall, 1995:196-202

Krige JEJ, Adams S, Simjee A. Amoebic liver abscess. In: Kirsch R, Robson S, Trey C, eds. *Diagnosis and management of liver disease.* London: Chapman and Hall, 1995:186-95

Krige JEJ, Terblanche J. Hepatic echinococcosis. In: Cameron JL, ed. *Current surgical therapy.* 6th ed. Baltimore, MA: Mosby, 1998:326-30

The picture of the trophozoite was supplied by David Mirecman, University of Utah.

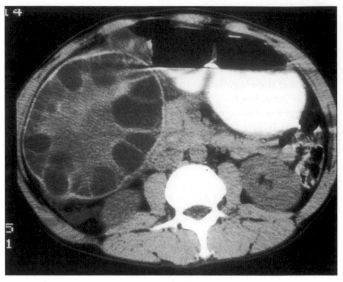

Figure 9.7 Computed tomogram showing hydatid cyst: daughter cysts containing hydatid larvae are visible within the main cyst

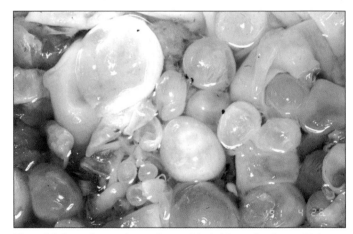

Figure 9.8 Operative specimen of opened hydatid cyst showing multiple daughter cysts

Summary points

- Most patients with pyogenic abscesses will require percutaneous drainage and antibiotics
- A cause can be identified in 85% of cases of liver abscess, most commonly gall stones, diverticulitis, or appendicitis
- Amoebic abscesses can be treated by metronidazole alone in 95% of cases
- Hydatid disease occurs throughout the world in sheep farming areas
- Symptomatic hydatid cysts should be surgically removed

10 Acute pancreatitis

I J Beckingham, P C Bornman

Acute pancreatitis is relatively common, with an annual incidence of 10-20/million population. In more than 80% of patients the disease is associated with alcohol or gall stones, although the ratio of these two causes has a wide geographical variation. Gallstone disease predominates in most UK centres by more than 2:1.

Pathogenesis and pathological processes

Apart from mechanical factors such as the passage of gall stones through the ampulla of Vater or cannulation at endoscopic retrograde cholangiopancreatography, little is known about how the disease process begins. What follows is also unclear, but proteolytic enzymes are thought to be activated while still within the pancreatic cells, setting off a local and systemic inflammatory cell response.

The process is self limiting in most cases and pathologically correlates with oedematous interstitial pancreatitis. In 15-20% of cases the process runs a fulminating course, most commonly within the first week. This is characterised by pancreatic necrosis and associated cytokine activation resulting in multiple organ dysfunction syndrome. The necrotic process mainly affects the peripancreatic tissue (mostly fat) and may spread extensively along the retroperitoneal space behind the colon and into the small bowel mesentery. The necrotic tissue can become infected, probably by translocation of bacteria from the gut.

Clinical presentation

Acute pancreatitis should always be considered in the differential diagnosis of patients with acute abdomen. The clinical presentation may vary considerably and is influenced by the aetiological factor, age, other associated illnesses, the stage of the disease, and the severity of the attack.

In alcohol induced pancreatitis symptoms usually begin 6-12 hours after an episode of binge drinking. Gall stones should be suspected in patients over 50 years of age (especially women), those who do not drink alcohol, and when the attack begins after a large meal. In patients with an alcohol history and proved gall stones it can be difficult to distinguish between the two causes. A serum alanine transaminase activity greater than three times above normal usually indicates that gall stones are the cause.

Patients usually have pain in the epigastrium that typically radiates through to the back. It is often associated with nausea and vomiting. Severe attacks often mimic other abdominal catastrophes such as perforated or ischaemic bowel and ruptured aortic aneurysm. Abdominal distension with or without a vague palpable epigastric mass is common in severe attacks. More rarely, patients develop discoloration in the lumbar regions and periumbilical area because of associated bleeding in the retroperitoneal space.

Acute pancreatitis may develop after cardiac or abdominal operations—for example, gastrectomy or biliary surgery—and the onset may be insidious with unexplained cardiorespiratory failure, fever, and ileus associated with minimal abdominal signs.

Box 10.1 Causes of acute pancreatitis

- Gallstones ⎤
- Alcohol ⎦ 80%
- Idiopathic: 10%
- Endoscopic retrograde cholangiopancreatography or sphincterectomy: 5%
- Miscellaneous: 5%
  Hyperlipidaemia
  Trauma
  Hyperparathyroidism
  Viral (mumps, Epstein-Barr virus, cytomegalovirus coxsackievirus)
  Drug induced (thiazide diuretics, angiotensin converting enzyme inhibitors, oestrogens, corticosteroids, azathioprine)
  Anatomical (pancreas divisum, annular pancreas)
  Parasites (*Ascaris lumbricoides*)

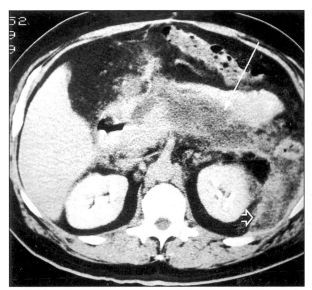

Figure 10.1 Computed tomogram showing extensive pancreatic necrosis (arrow) spreading into perinephric fat (open arrow head)

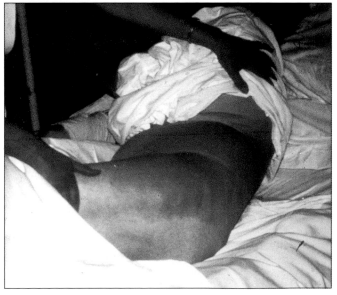

Figure 10.2 Discoloration of flank in patient with acute pancreatitis (Grey-Turner's sign)

33

Diagnosis

Pancreatitis is diagnosed on the basis of a combination of appropriate clinical features and a serum amylase activity over three times above normal (>330 U/l.). Lower activities do not rule out the diagnosis as serum amylase activity may reduce or normalise within the first 24-48 hours. Measurement of urinary amylase activity, which remains high for longer periods, may be helpful in this situation.

Although amylase activity may be raised in several other conditions with similar clinical signs (notably perforated peptic ulcer and ischaemic bowel), the increase is rarely more than three times above normal. Serum lipase measurement has a higher sensitivity and specificity, and now that simpler methods of measurement are available it is likely to become the preferred diagnostic test.

Clinical course

Whatever the underlying cause of pancreatitis, the clinical course is usually similar. The disease process is self limiting in 80% of cases, but in severe cases, there are usually three phases: local inflammation and necrosis, a systemic inflammatory response leading to multiple organ dysfunction syndrome during the first two weeks, and, finally, local complications such as the development of a pseudocyst or infection in the pancreatic and peripancreatic necrotic tissue.

Assessment of severity

Early identification of patients with a severe attack is important as they require urgent admission to a high dependency or intensive care unit. Initial predictors of a severe attack include first attack of alcohol induced pancreatitis, obesity, haemodynamic instability, and severe abdominal signs (severe tenderness and haemorrhage of the abdominal wall).

Several scoring systems have been developed to predict patients with mild or severe pancreatitis. The most widely used in the United Kingdom is the modified Glasgow system (Imrie), which has a sensitivity of 68% and a specificity of 84%. Other commonly used systems are Ranson's and the acute physiological and chronic health evaluation (APACHE II). Changes in C reactive protein concentration and APACHE II scores correlate well with the ongoing disease process.

Radiology

Chest and abdominal radiography are rarely diagnostic but are useful to exclude other acute abdominal conditions such as a perforated peptic ulcer. Abdominal ultrasonography is indicated at an early stage to identify gall stones and exclude biliary dilatation. The pancreas is visible in only 30-50% of patients because of the presence of bowel gas and obesity. When visible it appears oedematous and may be associated with fluid collections. Small gall stones may be missed during an acute episode, and if no cause is found patients should have repeat ultrasonography six to eight weeks after the attack.

In patients in whom a diagnosis of pancreatitis is uncertain, early computed tomography is useful to look for pancreatic and peripancreatic oedema and fluid collections. This avoids inappropriate diagnostic laparotomy. Patients who are thought to have severe pancreatitis or in whom treatment is failing to resolve symptoms should have contrast enhanced computed tomography after 72 hours to look for pancreatic necrosis.

Box 10.2 Differential diagnosis of acute pancreatitis

Mild attack
- Biliary colic or acute cholecystitis
- Complicated peptic ulcer disease
- Acute liver conditions
- Incomplete bowel obstruction
- Renal disease
- Lung disease (for example, pneumonia or pleurisy)

Severe attack
- Perforated or ischaemic bowel
- Ruptured aortic aneurysm
- Myocardial infarction

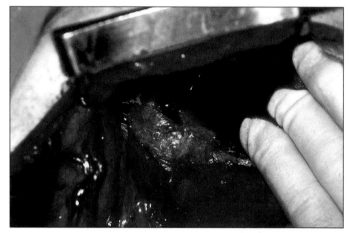

Figure 10.3 Removal of amylase-rich pericardial fluid from patient with acute pancreatitis

Box 10.3 Modified Glasgow criteria

- Age >55 years
- White cell count $>15\times10^9$/l
- Blood glucose >10 mmol/l
- Urea >16 mmol/l
- Arterial oxygen partial pressure <8.0 kPa
- Albumin <32 g/l
- Calcium <2.0 mmol/l
- Lactate dehydrogenase >600 U/l

Severe disease is present if ≥3 factors detected within 48 hours

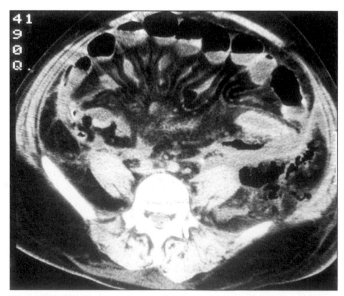

Figure 10.4 Computed tomogram showing extensive mesenteric oedema caused by retroperitoneal fluid due to acute pancreatitis

Treatment of acute attacks

Mild pancreatitis

Treatment of mild pancreatitis is supportive. Patients require hospital admission, where they should receive intravenous crystalloid fluids and appropriate analgesia and should stop all oral intake. Most patients will require opiate analgesia, and although this may cause spasm of the sphincter of Oddi, there is no evidence that this affects the outcome of the disease. A nasogastric tube may be helpful if vomiting is severe. Antibiotics are of no benefit in the absence of coexisting infections. Investigations are limited to the initial blood tests and ultrasonography when gall stones are suspected. Most patients will recover in 48-72 hours, and fluids can be restarted once abdominal pain and tenderness are resolving.

Severe pancreatitis

Patients with severe pancreatitis should be admitted to a high dependency or intensive care unit for close monitoring. Adequate resuscitation of hypovolaemic shock (which is often underestimated) remains the cornerstone of management, and patients often require surprisingly large volumes of fluids over the first 24-48 hours. Resuscitation is mainly with crystalloids, but colloids may be required to restore circulating volume. Progress is monitored by ensuring that urine output is adequate (>30 ml/h). Measurement of central venous or pulmonary arterial pressure may be required, particularly in patients with cardiorespiratory compromise. Patients who develop adult respiratory distress syndrome and renal failure require ventilation and dialysis.

The role of prophylactic antibiotics in severe pancreatitis remains unclear, but recent randomised trials have shown a marginal benefit with antibiotics that have good penetration into pancreatic tissue (such as high dose cefuroxime and imipenem).

Patients with severe gallstone pancreatitis and biliary sepsis or obstruction benefit from endoscopic retrograde cholangiopancreatography and removal of stones from the common bile duct within the first 48 hours of admission. However, the benefit of sphincterotomy is equivocal in patients without biliary obstruction.

Despite intensive search, no effective drug has been developed to prevent the development of severe pancreatitis. Several new drugs including antagonists of platelet activating factor (Lexipafant) and free radical scavengers that may limit propagation of the cytokine cascade hold theoretical promise, but initial clinical trials have been disappointing.

Patients who deteriorate despite maximum support pose a difficult management problem. The possibility of infection in the necrotic process should be considered, particularly when deterioration occurs after the first week. Infection can usually be confirmed by computed tomography guided fine needle aspiration. Patients with infected pancreatic necrosis have a 70% mortality and require surgical debridement (necrectomy). The role of necrectomy in patients without infection is unclear . Several new approaches are being investigated, including the use of minimally invasive necrectomy and lavage and the use of enteral rather than parenteral nutrition, which may reduce gut permeability and bacterial translocation and limit infection in the necrotic pancreas.

Prognosis

The overall mortality of patients with acute pancreatitis is 10-15% and has not changed in the past 20 years. The mortality of mild pancreatitis is below 5% compared with 20-25% in severe pancreatitis.

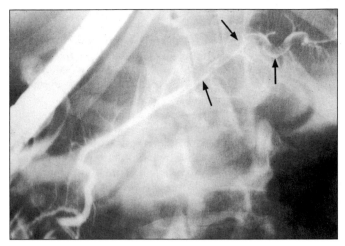

Figure 10.5 *Ascaris lumbricoides* in pancreatic duct: a rare cause of acute pancreatitis

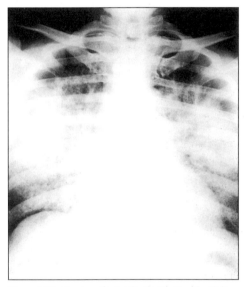

Figure 10.6 Chest radiograph of patient with adult respiratory distress syndrome as a complication of acute pancreatitis

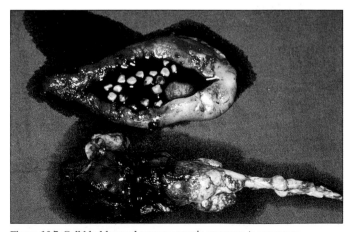

Figure 10.7 Gall bladder and severe necrotic pancreas (necrectomy specimen) removed from patient with acute pancreatitis induced by gall stones

Long term management

Patients with gall stones are best treated by laparoscopic cholecystectomy. This should ideally be done within the same hospital admission after the acute episode has settled to prevent recurrent attacks, which may be fatal. In high risk patients who are considered unfit for surgery, an endoscopic sphincterotomy will prevent most recurrent attacks.

Newer investigative techniques, including bile sampling and analysis and endoscopic ultrasonography, are showing that many patients with "idiopathic" pancreatitis have biliary microlithiasis due to cholesterol crystals, biliary sludge, or small stones that are missed by routine abdominal ultrasonography. Early results confirm that laparoscopic cholecystectomy is curative in most of these cases.

Further reading

Glazer G, Mann DV on behalf of working party of British Society of Gastroenterology. United Kingdom guidelines for the management of acute pancreatitis. *Gut* 1998;42(suppl 2)

A review of acute pancreatitis. *Eur J Gastroenterol Hepatol* 1997;9:1-120

Bradley EL. Complications of acute pancreatitis and their management. In: Trede M, Carter DC, Longmire WP, eds. *Surgery of the pancreas*. Edinburgh: Churchill Livingstone, 1997:245-62

Box 10.4 Key points

- Acute pancreatitis is a common cause of severe acute abdominal pain and gall stones are the commonest cause in the United Kingdom
- Severity scoring should be used to identify patients at greatest risk of complications
- Treatment is mainly supportive
- Patients with acute gallstone pancreatitis require early laparoscopic cholecystectomy once the attack has settled
- Biliary microlithiasis is increasingly recognised as a cause of "idiopathic" pancreatitis
- Mortality for acute pancreatitis is 10% overall but rises to 70% in patients with infected severe pancreatitis

11 Chronic pancreatitis

P C Bornman, I J Beckingham

Chronic pancreatitis has an annual incidence of about one person per 100 000 in the United Kingdom and a prevalence of 3/100 000. In temperate areas alcohol misuse accounts for most cases, and it mainly affects men aged 40-50 years. There is no uniform threshold for alcohol toxicity, but the quantity and duration of alcohol consumption correlates with the development of chronic pancreatitis. Little evidence exists, however, that either the type of alcohol or pattern of consumption is important. Interestingly, despite the common aetiology, concomitant cirrhosis and chronic pancreatitis is rare.

In a few tropical areas, most notably Kerala in southern India, malnutrition and ingestion of large quantities of cassava root are implicated in the aetiology. The disease affects men and women equally, with an incidence of up to 50/1000 population.

Natural course

Alcohol induced chronic pancreatitis usually follows a predictable course. In most cases the patient has been drinking heavily (150-200 mg alcohol/day) for over 10 years before symptoms develop. The first acute attack usually follows an episode of binge drinking, and with time these attacks may become more frequent until the pain becomes more persistent and severe. Pancreatic calcification occurs about 8-10 years after the first clinical presentation. Endocrine and exocrine dysfunction may also develop during this time, resulting in diabetes and steatorrhoea. There is an appreciable morbidity and mortality due to continued alcoholism and other diseases that are associated with poor living standards (carcinoma of the bronchus, tuberculosis, and suicide), and patients have an increased risk of developing pancreatic carcinoma. Overall, the life expectancy of patients with advanced disease is typically shortened by 10-20 years.

Symptoms and signs

The predominant symptom is severe dull epigastric pain radiating to the back, which may be partly relieved by leaning forward. The pain is often associated with nausea and vomiting, and epigastric tenderness is common. Patients often avoid eating because it precipitates pain. This leads to severe weight loss, particularly if patients have steatorrhoea.

Steatorrhoea presents as pale, loose, offensive stools that are difficult to flush away and, when severe, may cause incontinence. It occurs when over 90% of the functioning exocrine tissue is destroyed, resulting in low pancreatic lipase activity, malabsorption of fat, and excessive lipids in the stools.

One third of patients will develop overt diabetes mellitus, which is usually mild. Ketoacidosis is rare, but the diabetes is often "brittle," with patients having a tendency to develop hypoglycaemia due to a lack of glucagon. Hypoglycaemic coma is a common cause of death in patients who continue to drink or have had pancreatic resection.

Box 11.1 Aetiology of chronic pancreatitis

- Alcohol (80-90%)
- Nutritional (tropical Africa and Asia)
- Pancreatic duct obstruction (obstructive pancreatitis)
  Acute pancreatitis
  Pancreas divisum
- Cystic fibrosis
- Hereditary
- Idiopathic

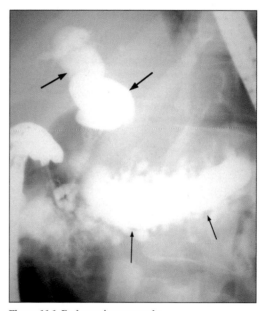

Figure 11.1 Endoscopic retrograde cholangiopancreatogram showing dilated common bile duct (thick arrow) and main pancreatic ducts (thin arrow) in patient with advanced chronic pancreatitis

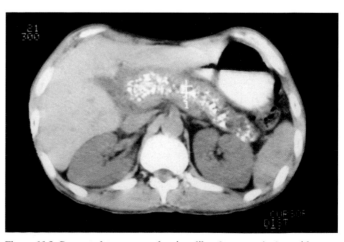

Figure 11.2 Computed tomogram showing dilated pancreatic duct with multiple calcified stones

Diagnosis

Early diagnosis of chronic pancreatitis is usually difficult. There are no reliable biochemical markers, and early parenchymal and ductal morphological changes may be hard to detect. The earliest signs (stubby changes of the side ducts) are usually seen on endoscopic retrograde cholangiopancreatography, but a normal appearance does not rule out the diagnosis. Tests of pancreatic function are cumbersome and seldom used to confirm the diagnosis. Thus, early diagnosis is often made by exclusion based on typical symptoms and a history of alcohol misuse.

In patients with more advanced disease, computed tomography shows an enlarged and irregular pancreas, dilated main pancreatic duct, intrapancreatic cysts, and calcification. Calcification may also be visible in plain abdominal radiographs. The classic changes seen on endoscopic retrograde cholangiopancreatography are irregular dilatation of the pancreatic duct with or without strictures, intrapancreatic stones, filling of cysts, and smooth common bile duct stricture.

Treatment

Treatment is focused on the management of acute attacks of pain and, in the long term, control of pain and the metabolic complications of diabetes mellitus and fat malabsorption. It is important to persuade the patient to abstain completely from alcohol. A team approach is essential for the successful long term management of complex cases.

Pain

Persistent or virtually permanent pain is the most difficult aspect of management and is often intractable. The cause of the pain is unknown. Free radical damage has been suggested as a cause, and treatment with micronutrient antioxidants (selenium, β carotene, methionine, and vitamins C and E) produces remission in some patients. However, further randomised trials are required to confirm the efficacy of this approach. In the later stages of disease pain may be caused by increased pancreatic ductal pressure due to obstruction, or by fibrosis trapping or damaging the nerves supplying the pancreas.

The mainstay of treatment remains abstinence from alcohol, but this does not always guarantee relief for patients with advanced disease. Analgesics should be prescribed with caution to prevent narcotic dependency as many patients have addictive personalities. Non-steroidal analgesics are the preferred treatment, but most patients with ongoing and relentless pain will ultimately require oral narcotic analgesics such as tilidine, tramadol, morphine, or meperidine. Slow release opioid patches (such as fentanyl) are increasingly used. Once this stage is reached patients should be referred to a specialist pain clinic.

Use of large doses of pancreatic extract to inhibit pancreatic secretion and reduce pain has unfortunately not lived up to expectations. Likewise coeliac plexus blocks have been disappointing, and it remains to be seen whether minimal access transthoracic splanchnicectomy will be effective.

Steatorrhoea

Steatorrhoea is treated with pancreatic replacements with the aim of controlling the loose stools and increasing the patient's weight. Pancreatic enzyme supplements are rapidly inactivated below pH5, and the most useful supplements are high concentration, enteric coated microspheres that prevent deactivation in the stomach—for example, Creon or Pancrease. A few patients also require H_2 receptor antagonists or dietary fat restriction.

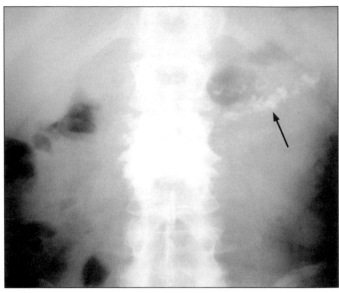

Figure 11.3 Plain abdominal radiograph showing multiple calcified stones within the pancreatic duct

Box 11.2 Team for management of complex cases
- General practitioner
- Physician or surgeon with an interest in chronic pancreatitis
- Dietician
- Clinical psychologist
- Chronic pain team
- Diabetologist

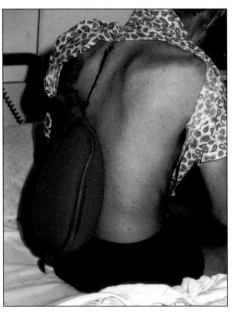

Figure 11.4 Patient using hot water bottle to relieve back pain due to chronic pancreatitis

Patients who do not gain weight despite adequate pancreatic replacement therapy and control of diabetes should be investigated for coexistent malignancy or tuberculosis.

Diabetes mellitus

The treatment of diabetes is influenced by the relative rarity of ketosis and angiopathy and by the hazards of potentially lethal insulin induced hypoglycaemia in patients who continue to drink alcohol or have had major pancreatic resection. It is thus important to undertreat rather than overtreat diabetes in these patients, and they should be referred to a diabetologist when early symptoms develop. Oral hypoglycaemic drugs should be used for as long as possible. Major pancreatic resection invariably results in the development of insulin dependent diabetes.

Endoscopic procedures

Endoscopic procedures to remove pancreatic duct stones, with or without extracorporeal lithotripsy and stenting of strictures, are useful both as a form of treatment and to help select patients suitable for surgical drainage of the pancreatic duct. However, few patients are suitable for these procedures, and they are available only in highly specialised centres.

Surgery

Surgery should be considered only after all forms of conservative treatment have been exhausted and when it is clear that the patient is at risk of becoming addicted to narcotics. Unless complications are present, the decision to operate is rarely easy, especially in patients who have already become dependent on narcotic analgesics.

The surgical strategy is largely governed by morphological changes to parenchymal and pancreatic ductal tissue. As much as possible of the normal upper gastrointestinal anatomy and pancreatic parenchyma should be preserved to avoid problems with diabetes mellitus and malabsorption of fat. The currently favoured operations are duodenal preserving resection of the pancreatic head (Beger procedure) and extended lateral pancreaticojejunostomy (Frey's procedure). More extensive resections such as Whipple's pancreatoduodenectomy and total pancreatectomy are occasionally required. The results of surgery are variable; most series report a beneficial outcome in 60-70% of cases at five years, but the benefits are often not sustainable in the long term. It is often difficult to determine whether failures are surgically related or due to narcotic addiction.

Complications of chronic pancreatitis

Pseudocysts

Pancreatic pseudocysts are localised collections of pancreatic fluid resulting from disruption of the duct or acinus. About 25% of patients with chronic pancreatitis will develop a pseudocyst. Pseudocysts in patients with chronic pancreatitis are less likely to resolve spontaneously than those developing after an acute attack, and patients will require some form of drainage procedure. Simple aspiration guided by ultrasonography is rarely successful in the long term, and most patients require internal drainage. Thin walled pseudocysts bulging into the stomach or duodenum can be drained endoscopically, with surgical drainage reserved for thick walled cysts and those not bulging into the bowel on endoscopy. Occasionally, rupture into the peritoneal cavity causes severe gross ascites or, via pleuroperitoneal connections, a pleural effusion.

Raised amylase activity in the ascitic or pleural fluid (usually > 20 000 iu/l) confirms the diagnosis. Patients should be given intravenous or jejunal enteral feeding to rest the bowel and

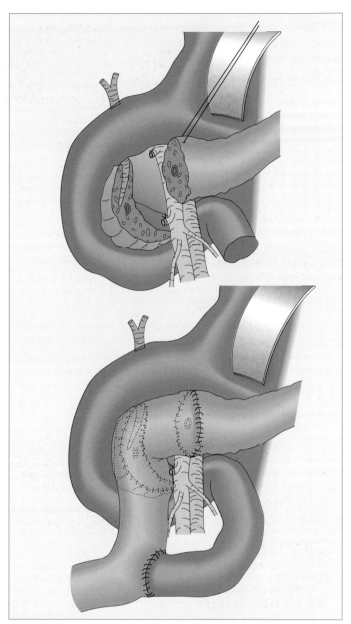

Figure 11.5 Duodenal preserving resection of the pancreatic head (Beger procedure). Top: pancreatic head resected. Bottom: reconstruction with jejunal Roux loop

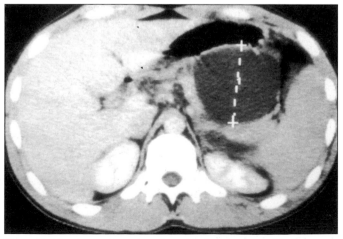

Figure 11.6 Large pseudocyst in patient with chronic pancreatitis. The cyst is thin walled and bulging into the stomach and is ideal for endoscopic drainage

minimise pancreatic stimulation, somatostatin infusion, and repeated aspiration. The cyst resolves in 70% of cases after two to three weeks. Persistent leaks require endoscopic stenting of the pancreatic duct or surgery to drain the site of leakage if it is proximal or resection if distal.

Biliary stricture

Stenosis of the bile duct resulting in persistent jaundice (more than a few weeks) is uncommon and usually secondary to pancreatic fibrosis. The duct should be drained surgically, and this is often done as part of surgery for associated pain or duodenal obstruction. Endoscopic stenting is not a long term solution, and is indicated only for relief of symptoms in high risk cases.

Gastroduodenal obstruction

Gastroduodenal obstruction is rare (1%) and usually due to pancreatic fibrosis in the second part of the duodenum. It is best treated by gastrojejunostomy.

Splenic vein thrombosis

Venous obstruction due to splenic vein thrombosis (segmental or sinistral hypertension) may cause splenomegaly and gastric varices. Most thrombi are asymptomatic but pose a severe risk if surgery is planned. Splenectomy is the best treatment for symptomatic cases.

Gastrointestinal bleeding

Gastrointestinal bleeding may be due to gastric varices, coexisting gastroduodenal disease, or pseudoaneurysms of the splenic artery, which occur in association with pseudocysts. Endoscopy is mandatory in these patients. Pseudoaneurysms are best treated by arterial embolisation or surgical ligation.

Further reading

Beckingham IJ, Krige JEJ, Bornman PC, Terblanche J. Endoscopic drainage of pancreatic pseudocysts. *Br J Surg* 1997;84:1638-45

Eckhauser FE, Colletti LM, Elta GH, Knol JA. Chronic pancreatitis. In: Pitt HA, Carr-Locke DL, Ferrucci JT, eds. *Hepatobiliary and pancreatic disease. The team approach to management.* Boston: Little, Brown, 1995:395-412

Misiewicz JJ, Pounder RE, Venables CW, eds. Chronic pancreatitis. In: *Diseases of the gut and pancreas.* Oxford: Blackwell Science, 1994:441-54

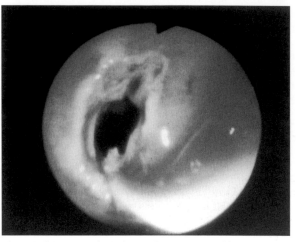

Figure 11.7 Endoscopic drainage of pseudocyst: sphincterotome is cutting a hole between stomach and pseudocyst wall

Summary points

- In most areas of the world alcohol is the main cause of chronic pancreatitis
- Early diagnosis is often difficult and relies on appropriate clinical history and imaging
- Stopping alcohol intake is essential to reduce attacks of pain, preserve pancreatic function, and aid management of complications
- Patients often require opiate analgesics, and pain is best managed in a multidisciplinary setting
- Surgery should be reserved for patients with intractable pain or with complications of chronic pancreatitis

12 Pancreatic tumours

P C Bornman, I J Beckingham

Neoplasms of the pancreas may originate from both exocrine and endocrine cells, and they vary from benign to highly malignant. Clinically, 90% of pancreatic tumours are malignant ductal adenocarcinomas, and most of this article concentrates on this disease.

Ductal adenocarcinoma

Incidence and prognosis
Carcinoma of the pancreas has become more common in most Western countries over the past three decades, and although there is evidence of plateauing in some countries such as the United States, it still ranks as the sixth commonest cause of cancer death in the United Kingdom. Most patients are over the age of 60 years (80%) and many will have concurrent medical illnesses that complicate management decisions, particularly because the median survival from diagnosis is less than six months.

Clinical presentation
Two thirds of pancreatic cancers develop in the head of the pancreas, and most patients present with progressive, obstructive jaundice with dark urine and pale stools. Pruritus, occurring as a result of biliary obstruction, is often troublesome and rarely responds to antihistamines. Back pain is a poor prognostic sign, often being associated with local invasion of tumours. Severe cachexia, as a result of increased energy expenditure mediated by the tumour, is also a poor prognostic indicator. Cachexia is the usual presenting symptom in patients with tumours of the body or tail of the pancreas.

Examination
The commonest sign is jaundice, with yellowing of the sclera and, once the bilirubin concentration exceeds 35 µmol/l, the skin. Many patients with high bilirubin concentrations will have skin scratches associated with pruritus. Patients with advanced disease have severe weight loss accompanied by muscle wasting and occasionally an enlarged supraclavicular lymph node. A palpable gall bladder suggests pancreatic malignancy, but it can be difficult to detect when displaced laterally or covered by an enlarged liver. The presence of ascites or a palpable epigastric mass usually indicates end stage disease. Full assessment of the patient's general fitness is essential to develop an individualised management plan.

Investigation
Because of the poor prognosis, care should be taken not to overinvestigate or embark on treatment strategies based on the unrealistic expectations of patients, their families, or the referring doctor. An increasing number of investigations are available, and the aim is to select patients who will not benefit from major resection by use of the fewest, least invasive, and least expensive means. The choice of investigation will vary according to local availability, particularly of newer investigations such as laparoscopic and endoscopic ultrasonography, and it remains to be seen if these techniques offer major advantages over the latest generation of computed tomography and magnetic resonance imaging scanners. Early cooperation between a gastroenterologist, radiologist, and

---

Box 12.1 Types of pancreatic neoplasms
- Benign exocrine
  Serous cyst adenoma
  Mucinous cyst adenoma
- Malignant exocrine
  Ductal adenocarcinoma
  Mucinous cyst adenocarcinoma
- Endocrine
  Gastrinoma
  Insulinoma
  Other

Box 12.2 Factors predicting poor prognosis
- Back pain
- Rapid weight loss
- Poor performance status—for example, World Health Organization or Karnofsky scoring systems
- Ascites and liver metastases
- High C reactive protein and low albumin concentrations

Box 12.3 Rarer presentations of pancreatic carcinoma
- Recurrent or atypical venous thromboses (thrombophlebitis migrans)
- Acute pancreatitis
- Late onset diabetes mellitus
- Upper gastrointestinal bleeding

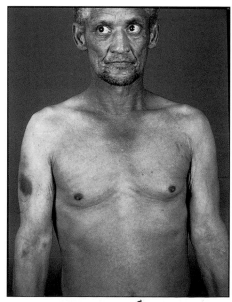

Figure 12.1 Patient with jaundice, bruising, and weight loss due to pancreatic carcinoma

surgeon should avoid inappropriate investigations and treatment that might interfere with patients' quality of life.

Endoscopic retrograde cholangiopancreatography is an important investigation in patients with obstructive jaundice. As well as showing biliary and pancreatic strictures, the pathology can be confirmed by taking brushings for cytology or biopsy specimens of the duct for histology. The technique can also be used to place a stent to relieve biliary obstruction. However, it is important not to use this approach before patients are properly selected for treatment.

The diagnosis can also be confirmed by fine needle aspiration guided by ultrasonography or computed tomography, but this investigation has a high rate of false negative results and is rarely necessary. Fine needle aspiration should be avoided in patients with potentially resectable tumours as it can cause seeding and spread of the tumour.

Treatment
Surgical resection does not improve survival in patients with locally advanced or metastatic disease. Tumour stage and the patient's fitness for major surgical resection are the main factors in determining optimal treatment.

Resectable tumours
Surgical resection, usually a pancreaticoduodenectomy (Whipple's procedure), is the only hope for cure. Less than 15% of tumours are suitable for resection. Very few tumours of the body and tail are resectable (3%) as patients usually present late with poorly defined symptoms.

The outcome of resection has been shown to be better in specialised pancreatobiliary centres that perform the procedure regularly than in small units. Mortality has fallen to 5-10% in dedicated units. The overall five year survival rate of 10-15% after resection remains disappointing, although survival is as high as 20-30% in some subgroups such as patients with small (<2 cm), node negative tumours. Furthermore, the median survival of patients who have resection is 18 months compared with six months for patients without metastatic disease who do not have resection.

Preoperative biliary drainage remains controversial. The reduced complications from resolution of jaundice are offset by more inflammatory tissue at surgery and higher rates of biliary sepsis after stenting. Ideally patients with minimal jaundice should be operated on without stenting whereas those with higher bilirubin concentrations (>100 µmol/l) probably benefit from endoscopic stenting and reduction of bilirubin concentrations before surgery.

Locally advanced disease
Several options are available for the 65% of patients who have locally advanced disease. These depend on factors such as age, disease stage, and the patient's fitness. Endoscopic insertion of a plastic or metal wall stent relieves jaundice in most patients. Plastic stents are cheaper but have a median half life of three to four months compared with six months for metal stents. Blockage of a stent results in rigors and jaundice, and patients should be given antibiotics and have the stent replaced.

Surgical exploration and bypass should be used in patients who are predicted to survive longer than six months, in whom it is not certain that the tumour cannot be resected, in areas with limited access to endoscopic retrograde cholangiopancreatography, or with recurrent stent blockage or obstruction of the gastric outlet. Surgical bypass (open or laparoscopic) now has a low mortality and has the advantage of long term palliation of jaundice with a low risk of recurrence.

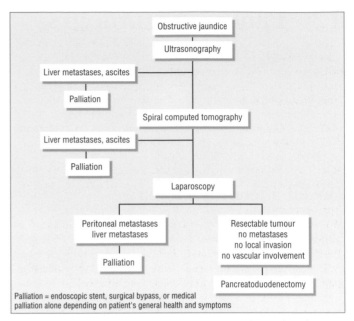

Figure 12.2 Investigation and management of pancreatic ductal carcinoma

Table 12.1 Treatment of pancreatic ductal carcinoma

Fitness of patient	Tumour stage		
	Resectable	Locally advanced	Metatstatic
Low risk	Pancreatoduodectomy	Surgical bypass or endoscopic stent	Palliative care +/− endoscopic stent
High risk	Endoscopic stent	Endoscopic stent	Palliative care

Box 12.4 Tumours suitable for resection
- <4 cm in diameter
- Confined to pancreas
- No local invasion or metastases

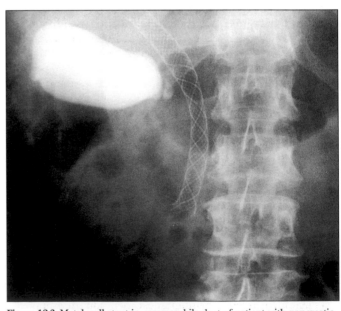

Figure 12.3 Metal wall stent in common bile duct of patient with pancreatic carcinoma. (Note contrast in gall bladder from endoscopic retrograde cholangiopancreatography)

Metastatic disease

Patients with metastatic disease are often cachectic and rarely survive more than a few weeks. Treatment should focus on alleviation of pain and improving quality of life with input from palliative care teams. Patients with less advanced metastatic disease may require endoscopic stenting, especially if they have intractable pruritus.

Radiotherapy and chemotherapy

Despite numerous trials, radiotherapy with or without chemotherapy has not been shown to prolong survival. The search for new chemotherapeutic and immunotherapeutic drugs continues, but they currently have little role outside clinical trials.

Symptom control

A liberal policy of pain control with paracetamol, non-steroidal anti-inflammatory drugs, and opiate analgesics should be followed. In difficult cases and when increasingly large doses of opiates are required, patients should be referred to a specialist pain clinic for consideration of coeliac plexus block or thoracoscopic splanchnicectomy. Early referral to the palliative care team and Macmillan nurses, who can bridge the gap between hospital and community care, is beneficial.

Cachexia is an important cause of disability in many patients. Nutritional supplementation rarely combats weight loss, and pancreatic replacement therapy is also of doubtful benefit. Encouraging results have recently been reported with polyunsaturated fatty acids (fish oil) and non-steroidal anti-inflammatories, which seem to inhibit the inflammatory response provoked by the tumour and reduce the speed of weight loss with some survival benefit. Impaired gastric emptying is generally underdiagnosed and may be functional or mechanical in origin.

Cystic tumours

These rare tumours (1% of all pancreatic neoplasms) are mostly benign, but the mucinous type (about 50%) is premalignant. They are important because they occur predominantly in young women and usually have a good prognosis when resected. Cystic tumours may be mistaken for benign pseudocysts, although they can usually be differentiated on the basis of history and computed tomographic findings (tumours have septa within the cyst and calcification of the rim of the cyst wall without calcification in the rest of the pancreas). If the diagnosis is in doubt, surgical resection with frozen section at the time of definitive surgery is the optimal management.

Endocrine tumours

Tumours arising from the islets of Langerhans can produce high concentrations of the hormones normally produced by the islets (insulin, glucagon, somatostatin, etc) or non-pancreatic hormones (such as gastrin or vasoactive peptide). Endocrine tumours are rare, with an incidence of around 1-2 per million population. The commonest forms are gastrinoma and insulinoma. They may be sporadic or occur as part of the multiple endocrine neoplasia syndrome, when they are associated with tumours of the pituitary, parathyroid, thyroid, and adrenal glands.

Patients usually present with a clinical syndrome produced by hormonal excess, typically of a single peptide. With the exception of insulinomas most endocrine tumours are malignant. Treatment is by surgical excision, and survival is generally good; 10 year survival rates for patients with malignant lesions are around 50%.

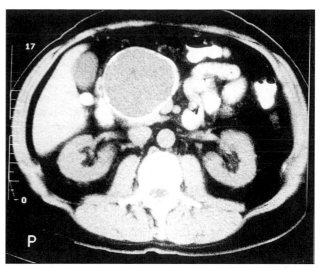

Figure 12.4 Cystic tumour in head of pancreas with calcified rim

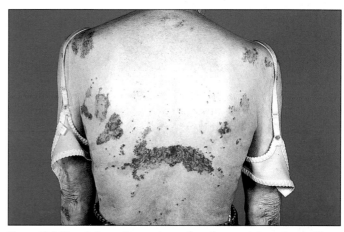

Figure 12.5 Necrolytic erythema migrans is pathognomic in patients with glucagonoma

---

Summary points

- 6000 people die from pancreatic cancer each year in the United Kingdom
- Presentation is usually with painless insidious jaundice
- Median survival from diagnosis is less than six months
- Less than 15% of all pancreatic tumours are resectable, and five year survival after resection is 10-15%
- Endoscopic retrograde cholangiopancreatography and surgical biliary drainage offer good palliation of jaundice
- Cystic and endocrine pancreatic tumours are uncommon but have a better prognosis

---

Further reading

Trede M, Carter DC. Surgical options for pancreatic cancer. In: *Surgery of the pancreas.* Edinburgh: Churchill Livingstone, 1997:383-515
Cameron JL, Grochow LB, Milligan FD, Venbrux AC. Pancreatic cancer. In: Pitt HA, Carr-Locke DL, Ferrucci JT, eds. *Hepatobiliary and pancreatic disease—the team approach to management.* Boston: Little Brown, 1995:475-86
Cotton P, Williams C. ERCP and therapy. In: *Practical gastrointestinal endoscopy.* Oxford: Blackwell Science, 1996:167-86

13 Liver and pancreatic trauma

I J Beckingham, J E J Krige

The liver is the most commonly injured solid intra-abdominal organ, but injuries to the pancreas are fairly rare. The primary goal in the treatment of severe abdominal injuries is to preserve life, and management is divided into four sequential phases: resuscitation, evaluation, initial management, and definitive treatment.

Liver trauma

Liver trauma constitutes a broad spectrum of injuries. The magnitude of the injury, the management requirements, and the complexity of the surgical repair are determined by the extent, anatomical location, and mechanism of injury. Blunt liver trauma is usually due to road traffic accidents, assaults, or falls from heights, and results in deceleration injuries with lacerations of liver tissue from shearing stresses. High velocity projectiles, close range shotgun injuries, and crushing blunt trauma cause fragmentation of the hepatic parenchyma with laceration of vessels and massive intraperitoneal haemorrhage. Penetrating injuries such as stab or gunshot wounds cause bleeding without much devitalisation of the liver parenchyma.

Resuscitation

Resuscitation follows standard advanced trauma life support principles: maintenance of a clear airway, urgent fluid resuscitation, ventilatory and circulatory support, and control of bleeding. Effective venous access should be obtained and volume replacement started immediately. The patient's blood is grouped and crossmatched, and blood samples should be sent for urgent analysis of haemoglobin concentration, white cell count, blood gas pressures, and urea, creatinine, and electrolyte concentrations. Patients should also have a nasogastric tube and urinary catheter inserted.

A liver injury should be suspected in patients with evidence of blunt trauma or knife or gunshot wounds to the right upper quadrant or epigastrium. Occasionally physical signs may be minimal, and gunshot entry and exit wounds can be deceptively distant from the liver. Diagnosis may be difficult in patients who are not fully conscious or have head or spinal cord injuries. The insidious onset of shock in a multiply injured or unconscious patient can easily be missed.

Evaluation

The most important decision after initial resuscitation is whether urgent surgery is needed. Patients who respond to fluid resuscitation and remain stable can be observed closely, investigated, and re-evaluated. Patients who remain shocked after 3 litres of intravenous fluid usually have continued bleeding and require urgent laparotomy. Surgery should not be delayed to obtain the results of special investigations.

Computed tomography of the abdomen is useful in haemodynamically stable patients suspected of having a major liver injury. Patients with large intrahepatic haematomas or limited capsular tears who have small volumes of blood in the peritoneal cavity can be treated non-operatively. They must, however, be observed carefully and have repeated physical examination.

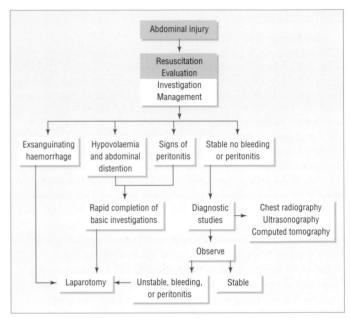

Figure 13.1 Management of major abdominal trauma

Box 13.1 Clinical features of serious liver injury

- Hypovolaemic shock:
  - Hypotension
  - Tachycardia
  - Decreased urine output
  - Low central venous pressure
- Abdominal distension

Box 13.2 Criteria for non-operative management of liver injuries

- Haemodynamically stable after resuscitation
- No persistent or increasing abdominal pain or tenderness
- No other peritoneal injuries that require laparotomy
- < 4 units of blood transfusion required
- Haemoperitoneum <500 ml on computed tomography
- Simple hepatic parenchymal laceration or intrahepatic haematoma on computed tomography

---

Box 13.3 Indications for laparotomy

- Stab or gunshot wounds that have penetrated the abdomen
- Signs of peritonitis
- Unexplained shock
- Evisceration
- Uncontrolled haemorrhage
- Clinical deterioration during observation

Surgical management

Most liver injuries are simple and can be treated relatively easily. Complex lesions need to be diagnosed early and may require major surgery by an experienced hepatobiliary surgeon.

Operative approach

Patients should be prepared from the sternal notch to the pubis so that the incision can be extended into the chest if more proximal control of the vena cava or aorta is needed. A midline incision is used, and the first step is to remove blood and clots and control active bleeding from liver lacerations by packing. Care should be taken to avoid sustained periods of hypotension, and it is important to restore the patient's circulating blood volume during surgery. Any perforations in the bowel should be rapidly sutured to minimise contamination.

Most liver injuries have stopped bleeding spontaneously by the time of surgery. These wounds do not require suturing but should be drained to prevent bile collections. Liver bleeding can usually be stopped by compressing the liver with abdominal packs while experienced surgical and anaesthetic help is summoned.

If visibility is obscured by continued bleeding, the hepatic artery and portal vein should be temporarily clamped with a vascular clamp to allow accurate identification of the site of bleeding. If bleeding cannot be stopped the area should be packed; absorbable gauze mesh can be wrapped around an injured lobe and sutured to maintain pressure and tamponade bleeding. The abdomen is then closed without drainage and the packing removed under general anaesthesia two to three days later. Packing is also used if a coagulopathy develops or to allow the patient to be transferred to a tertiary referral unit for definitive management.

Patients with blunt injuries associated with substantial amounts of parenchymal destruction may require resectional debridement. Rarely, a severe crushing injury necessitates a formal hepatic lobectomy. The most difficult problems are lacerations of the vena cava and major hepatic veins behind the liver because temporary clamping of the inflow vessels does not slow blood loss from hepatic veins. Advanced operative techniques including total hepatic vascular isolation by clamping the portal vein and the vena cava above and below the liver or lobectomy may be required.

Postoperative complications

Rebleeding from the injury, bile leaks, ischaemic segments of liver, and infected fluid collections are the main postoperative complications associated with liver trauma. Angiography (with selective embolisation) is useful if recurrent arterial bleeding or haemobilia occur. Computed tomography is used to define intra-abdominal collections, which are best drained by ultrasound guided needle aspiration or a percutaneous catheter. Subhepatic sepsis develops in about a fifth of cases and is usually related to bile leaks, ischaemic tissue, undrained collections, or bowel injury. The site of bile leaks is best identified by endoscopic retrograde cholangiopancreatography and treated by endoscopic sphincterotomy or stenting, or both.

Prognosis

The overall mortality after liver injury is 10-15% and depends largely on the type of injury and the extent of injury to other organs. Only 1% of penetrating civilian wounds are lethal, whereas the mortality after blunt trauma exceeds 20%. The mortality after blunt hepatic injury is 10% when only the liver is injured. If three major organs are injured, however, mortality approaches 70%. Bleeding causes more than half of the deaths.

> **The priorities of surgery are to stop haemorrhage, remove dead or devitalised liver tissue, and ligate or repair damaged blood vessels and bile ducts.**

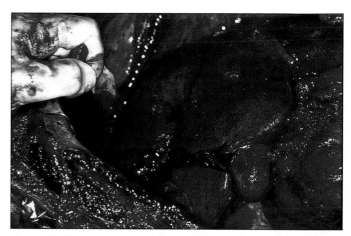

Figure 13.2 Stellate fracture of right lobe of liver

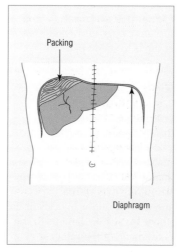
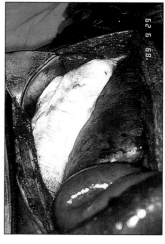

Figure 13.3 Packing of bleeding liver

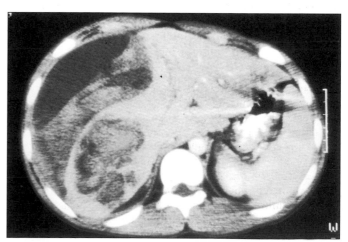

Figure 13.4 Large intrahepatic haematoma in patient with blunt trauma

Pancreatic trauma

Injuries to the pancreas are uncommon and account for 1-4% of severe abdominal injuries. Most pancreatic injuries occur in young men. Blunt trauma to the pancreas and duodenum usually results from road traffic accidents, when an unrestrained driver is thrown on to the steering wheel. Handlebars may inflict similar injuries to motorcyclists or children on bicycles. Deceleration injury during blunt trauma to the epigastrium may transect the neck of the pancreas over the vertebral bodies. The deep location of the pancreas means that considerable force is needed to cause an injury, and patients often have damage to surrounding organs, including the liver, spleen, stomach, duodenum, and colon. Penetrating injuries may also damage the portal vein or inferior vena cava.

Diagnosis

Blunt trauma to the pancreas may be clinically occult and parenchymal and duct injury may not be recognised during initial evaluation or even surgery. A high index of suspicion is therefore necessary in patients with severe upper abdominal injuries. Abdominal radiographs may show retroperitoneal air and a ruptured duodenum. Serum amylase activity is a poor indicator. It can be normal in patients with severe pancreatic damage and increased in patients with no demonstrable injury to the pancreas. Contrast enhanced computed tomography is the best investigation. Features of pancreatic injury include pancreatic oedema or swelling and fluid collections within or behind the peritoneum or in the lesser peritoneal sac. Endoscopic retrograde cholangiopancreatography can be use to assess the integrity of the main ducts in stable patients.

Intraoperative evaluation

Pancreatic injury is usually diagnosed at laparotomy. The injury may be obvious in patients with a major fracture of the body or neck of the pancreas or associated duodenal injury. Other clues to pancreatic injury are retroperitoneal bile staining, fat necrosis, peripancreatic oedema, or subcapsular haematoma. The pancreas should be fully mobilised and exposed to rule out a duct injury. Failure to detect a major injury to the pancreatic duct is an important cause of postoperative morbidity.

Haemodynamically stable patients with minor injuries of the body or tail of the pancreas who have no visible damage to the duct can be managed by external drainage of the injury site with soft silastic drains. Major injuries of the body and tail of the pancreas that affect the duct should be treated by distal pancreatectomy. Patients with injuries to the head of the pancreas without devitalisation of pancreatic tissue can be managed by external drainage provided that any associated duodenal injury is amenable to simple repair.

Pancreatoduodenectomy as a primary procedure is restricted to stabilised patients with disruption of the ampulla of Vater or major devitalising injuries of the pancreatic head and duodenum. Injuries of this severity occur after blunt trauma or gunshot wounds but are uncommon with stab wounds.

Complications

Pancreatic fistulas are the most common complication and generally close spontaneously. However, if a serious duct injury is present, a chronic fistula may develop and require surgical intervention. Pseudocysts that follow pancreatic injury are usually the result of inadequate drainage of pancreatic injury or failure to recognise a major ductal injury. They can be treated by percutaneous drainage guided by ultrasonography or computed tomography if the pancreatic injury was minor. However, patients who have major duct injury may require internal drainage or pancreatic resection.

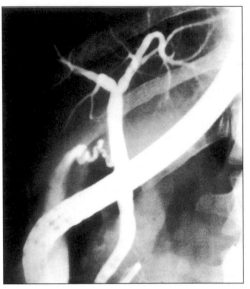

Figure 13.5 Endoscopic retrograde cholangiopancreatograph showing injury to pancreatic duct with obstruction in the pancreatic neck

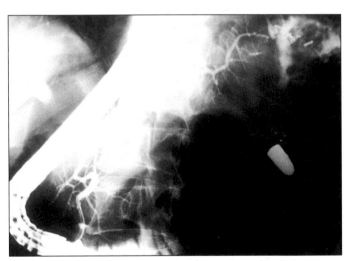

Figure 13.6 Pancreatic leak caused by a gunshot wound. The bullet is also visible

---

Box 13.4 Complications associated with pancreatic trauma

- Intra-abdominal abscess
- Wound infection
- Pancreatic fistula
- Pseudocyst
- Pancreatic abscess or ascites
- Acute or chronic pancreatitis

Further reading

Feliciano DV, Lewis CA. Hepatic trauma. In: Pitt H, Carr-Locke DL, Ferrucci R, eds. *Hepatobiliary and pancreatic disease*. Boston: Little, Brown, 1994:107-24

Pachter HL, Hofsetter SR. The current status of nonoperative management of adult blunt hepatic injuries. *Am J Surg* 1995;169:442-54.

Krige JEJ, Bornman PC, Beningfield SJ, Funnell I. Pancreatic trauma. In: Pitt H, Carr-Locke DL, Ferrucci R, eds. *Hepatobiliary and pancreatic disease*. Boston: Little, Brown, 1994:421-36

14 Transplantation of the liver and pancreas

K R Prasad, J P A Lodge

Liver transplantation is carried out for many chronic liver diseases and for fulminant hepatic failure. The United Kingdom has seven liver transplantation units, which perform 600-700 transplantations a year. Activity is limited by availability of donor organs, and there are around 200 patients waiting for a liver transplant at any one time. Transplantation of the pancreas is less well established. The pancreas is usually transplanted together with a kidney in patients with end stage diabetes mellitus and renal failure. Worldwide, around 1000 patients (mainly in the United States) receive a pancreatic transplant each year. Only 20-30 a year are transplanted in the United Kingdom.

Liver transplantation

Indications and contraindications
Hepatocellular carcinoma complicates many chronic liver diseases, and a small tumour is not a contraindication to transplantaton because tumour recurrence is uncommon in these patients. However, most patients with large (>5 cm) or multiple hepatomas or most other types of cancer are not considered for transplantation as tumours recur rapidly. Patients with certain rare tumours, such as liver metastases from neuroendocrine disease and sarcomas, can do well for several years. Contraindications to liver transplantation include extrahepatic malignancy, severe cardiopulmonary disease, systemic sepsis, and an inability to comply with regular drug treatment.

Timing and selection of patients for transplantation
The preoperative status of the patient is one of the most important factors predicting the outcome after transplantation. Patients with chronic liver disease and signs of decompensation should be assessed for transplantation before they become critically ill. In certain diseases, such as primary biliary cirrhosis, quality of life issues may form the basis for indication for transplantation. For example, chronic lack of energy can be debilitating in patients with biliary cirrhosis.

Acute liver failure and timing of transplantation
Liver transplantation greatly improves the prognosis of patients with fulminant liver failure. In the United Kingdom paracetamol overdose is now the commonest cause of acute liver failure, followed by seronegative (non-A, non-B, non-C) hepatitis.

The mortality from fulminant liver failure can be as high as 90%, whereas one year survival after urgent transplantation is often above 70%. In the United Kingdom, criteria developed at King's College Hospital are used for listing patients for "super urgent" transplantation. This scheme relies on cooperation between the liver transplantation centres to allow transplantation within 48 hours of listing whenever possible.

Surgical procedure
Before organs are removed an exploratory laparotomy is done on the donor to rule out any disease process (such as unexpected carcinoma) that may preclude organ donation. The major vessels are then dissected and blood flow controlled in preparation for hypothermic perfusion with a cold preservation solution. University of Wisconsin preservation solution is used most widely. It can preserve the liver adequately for about 13 hours, with acceptable results up to 24 hours.

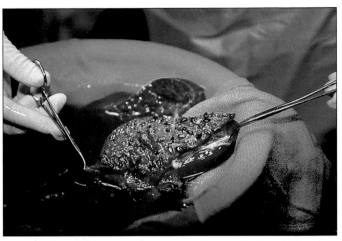

Figure 14.1 Donor liver from adult cut down for insertion into child recipient

---

Box 14.1 Common indications for liver transplantation
- Primary biliary cirrhosis
- Primary sclerosing cholangitis
- Cryptogenic cirrhosis
- Chronic active hepatitis (usually secondary to hepatitis B and C)
- Alcoholic liver disease (after a period of abstinence)

Box 14.2 Signs of decompensation in chronic liver disease
- Tiredness
- Ascites
- Encephalopathy
- Peripheral oedema
- Jaundice (not always a feature)
- Spontaneous bacterial peritonitis—abdominal pain (a late sign)
- Bleeding oesophageal or gastric varices
- Low albumin concentration
- Raised prothrombin time

Box 14.3 Paracetamol overdose
- Causes death by acute liver failure
- Renal failure develops as a hepatorenal syndrome and by acute tubular necrosis but is usually recoverable
- Early deaths usually result from raised intracranial pressure, and comatose patients require monitoring in an intensive care unit
- Death in later stages can occur from multiorgan failure and systemic sepsis
- If the patient survives without transplantation, the liver will recover without the development of cirrhosis

---

The donor organ is usually procured as part of a multiorgan retrieval from a heart beating, brain dead patient

Hepatectomy in the organ recipient is the most difficult part of the operation as the patient is at risk of developing a serious haemorrhage due to a combination of portal hypertension, defective clotting, and fibrinolysis. Improvements in surgical technique and anaesthesia have resulted in large reductions in blood loss, and the average requirement for transfusion is now four units of blood. At reimplantation, the suprahepatic and infrahepatic inferior vena cava and the portal vein are anastomosed and the organ is reperfused with blood. This is followed by reconstruction of the hepatic artery and bile duct.

Postoperative management
Patients are usually managed in an intensive care unit for the first 12-24 hours after surgery. Enteral feeding is restarted as early as possible, and liver function tests are done daily. Immunosuppressive protocols usually include a combination of cyclosporin or tacrolimus together with azathioprine or mycophenolate mofetil and prednisolone. The dose of steroids is rapidly tapered off, and they can often be stopped after two to three months. The doses of cyclosporin or tacrolimus are reduced gradually during the first year (during which pregnancy should be avoided) and continued at much lower levels for life.

Acute rejection occurs in about half of patients, but this is easily treated in most cases with extra steroids or by altering the drug regimen. Despite routine use of prophylactic treatment against bacterial, viral, and fungal pathogens, infections remain a major cause of morbidity. The side effects of the drugs are usually well controlled before the patient leaves hospital about two weeks after surgery.

At discharge, patients need to be familiarised with the drug regimen and side effects and educated about the warning signs of rejection and infection. Patients are usually followed up weekly for the first three months and then at gradually increasing intervals thereafter.

Results
The five year survival is 60-90%, depending on the primary disease and the clinical state of the patient before transplantation. The newer antiviral drugs plus the preoperative and postoperative adjuvant therapies for malignancies should lead to further improvements in survival. Although alcoholic liver disease remains a controversial indication for transplantation, carefully selected patients do well.

After successful transplantation patients have a greatly improved lifestyle and are often able to return to work and normal social activities. However, some patients experience medical and social problems. Drug compliance is one of the biggest problems after all types of organ transplantation. Poor compliance leads to chronic rejection and loss of the graft.

An extensive network of support services is available to help liver transplant patients. These include the transplant team, referring physician, general practitioner, social services, and local liver patient support groups. Shared care protocols operate in most regions, with most patients cared for primarily by their general practitioner and a gastroenterologist at their local hospital. The mainstay of follow up is regular liver function tests to detect any dysfunction of the transplant. Regular discussion of concerns with the transplant team is essential, and many problems can be sorted out by telephone.

Paediatric liver transplantation
In children, the most common indication for liver transplantation is biliary atresia, often after failure to respond to a portoenterostomy. Most children who need a liver transplant are young (under 3 years) and small (< 20 kg). Size matched donors are in short supply, and reduced size ("cut down") and

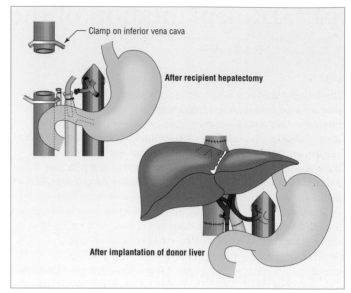

Figure 14.2 Implantation of liver transplant after hepatectomy

Table 14.1 Side effects of immunosuppresive drugs

Drug	Side effect	Monitoring
Cyclosporin	Neurotoxicity, nephrotoxicity, hypertension, hirsutism, gum hyperplasia, diabetes	Drug concentrations
Tacrolimus	Nephrotoxicity, neurotoxicity, hair loss, hypertension, diabetes	Drug concentrations
Azathioprine	Leucopenia, hair loss	White blood cell count
Mycophenolate mofetil	Gastrointestinal upset, leucopenia	White blood cell count and gastrointestinal symptoms
Steroids	Osteoporosis, diabetes, cushingoid face, hypertension	Symptoms
General	Infections, malignancy	Liver and renal function tests, regular follow up, and high index of suspicion

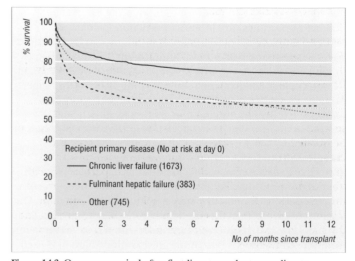

Figure 14.3 One year survival after first liver transplant according to primary disease, United Kingdom 1985-94

split (where one liver is split between two recipients) liver techniques have been used to overcome this problem. Donation of the left lobe of the liver by a living relative is also possible.

Pancreatic transplantation

The goals of transplantation of the pancreas are to eliminate the morbidity associated with labile blood glucose concentrations, stabilise or improve secondary diabetic complications, and improve the quality of life of patients with diabetes mellitus by restoring normal glucose metabolism. The stabilisation of diabetic control, the avoidance of exogenous insulin, and the ability to return to a normal diet for the first time since childhood are indisputable benefits of this procedure.

The selection of recipients for pancreatic transplantation is crucial. The magnitude of the surgery and need for long term immunosuppression means that whole organ transplantation is currently reserved for patients with end stage disease. Recipients are typically young (<50 years) with type 1 diabetes and end stage renal disease but without untreatable peripheral vascular or coronary artery disease. Simultaneous transplantation of the pancreas and kidney is the commonest procedure. Separate transplantation of the pancreas after kidney transplantation increases the chances of getting a good HLA matching for the kidney and allows a kidney to be donated by a living relative. The presence of immunosuppression at the time of implantation of the pancreas is also advantageous. The transplanted pancreas is usually placed in the pelvis and anastamosed to the iliac vessels, with the pancreatic duct anastomosed to the bladder or a loop of small bowel.

First year mortality is 3-10% in large units, with most deaths due to overwhelming sepsis. Transplant survival is 86% for the kidney and 70% for the pancreas. Successful transplantation greatly improves quality of life, and most patients are fully rehabilitated. Glucose homoeostasis seems to be excellent after pancreatic transplantation. Patients can stop exogenous insulin treatment and have normal glycated haemoglobin concentrations and glucose tolerance test results within three months of transplantation.

The long term effect on diabetic complications will not be known for several years, but recent results are encouraging. Evidence that diabetic nephropathy does not recur in the kidney transplant is accumulating, but there is no evidence for amelioration of established glomerular lesions in native kidneys. Improvements in autonomic and peripheral neuropathy have been documented. Further studies are needed to examine the potential for reducing the rate of progression of retinopathy and macrovascular disease.

Isolated pancreatic islet transplantation

A more logical approach is to attempt to prevent the development of the irreversible complications of diabetes by improving blood glucose metabolism at an early stage. Transplantation of pancreatic islet cells has been studied extensively as an alternative to whole organ grafting and has several theoretical and practical advantages. Pancreatic islets can be isolated by using collagenase digestion to separate the endocrine from the exocrine tissues and purified by density gradient separation. Some difficulties remain, particularly with the purification stage. The islets are injected into the recipient liver via the portal vein or by subcapsular injection into the kidney or spleen. Rejection of the islets remains a problem, and the success rates of this type of transplantation have been poor in the clinical setting.

> **The shortage of child liver donors has been partly resolved by using smaller sections of adult livers, usually the left lobe**

Table 14.2 Types of pancreatic transplantation

Type	Indication
Simultaneous pancreas and kidney transplant (SPK)	Diabetic renal failure
Pancreas after kidney transplant (PAK)	After successful kidney transplant
Pancreas transplant alone (PTA)	Prerenal failure, unstable diabetic control, severe neuropathy
Segmental (transplantation of pancreatic tail)	Applicable to live donation
Multivisceral (pancreas transplanted with liver and sometimes small bowel)	For example, extensive abdominal tumour
Isolated pancreatic islets	The future solution?

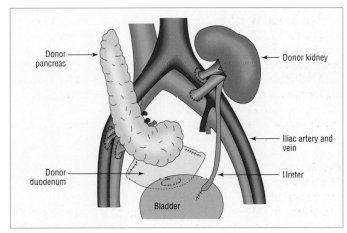

Figure 14.4 Simultaneous transplantation of pancreas and kidney with bladder drainage

Summary points

- Hepatitis C cirrhosis is the commonest worldwide indication for liver transplantation
- Alcoholic liver disease remains a controversial indication for liver transplantation but carefully selected patients do well
- Patients with chronic liver disease and signs of decompensation should be assessed for transplantation before they become critically ill
- Drug compliance is an important problem, with poor compliance leading to chronic rejection and graft loss
- Paracetamol overdose is the commonest cause of acute liver failure in the United Kingdom and accounts for 5% of all liver transplants in Britain
- Pancreas transplantation is most commonly performed for patients with end stage diabetes mellitus and renal failure

The photo of donor liver was obtained from J L Martha/Science Photo Library.

Index

Index

Index

adenocarcinomas 41–3
  chronic pancreatitis 38
  stones 39
  trauma 36
pancreatic enzyme supplements 38
pancreatic head, duodenal preserving
  resection (Beger procedure) 39
pancreaticoduodenectomy 39, 42, 46
pancreaticojejunostomy 39
pancreatitis, acute 33–6
  alcohol-induced 33, 34
  biliary microlithiasis 36
  biliary sepsis 35
  common bile duct stones 8
  gallstones 6, 33, 34, 35, 36
  hepatitis B infection 9
  necrectomy 35
  scoring systems 34
pancreatitis, chronic 1, 37–40
  alcohol misuse 37, 38
  calcification 3, 37, 38
  pain 38
  pancreatic carcinoma 37
  pseudocysts 39–40
  splenic vein thrombosis 40
  steatorrhoea 37, 38
pancreatitis, oedematous interstitial 33
paracentesis 23
  diagnostic 22, 24
paracetamol poisoning 16, 43, 47
parathyroid tumours 43
penicillamine 16
penicillin 30
percutaneous transhepatic cholangiography
  (PTC) 3, 17
pericarditis 9
perinuclear antineutrophil cytoplasmic
  antibody 17
peripancreatic tissue
  necrosis 33, 34
  oedema 46
peritoneovenous shunts 23
peritonitis
  amoebic 31
  spontaneous bacterial 24
phosphorus 2
pituitary tumours 43
plasma proteins 2–3
pleural effusion 9, 31, 39
polycystic liver disease 25
polymyalgia 15
polyneuritis 9
polyunsaturated fatty acids 43
portal hypertension 18–24
  ascites 18, 22–3
  cirrhosis 18
  hepatic encephalopathy 23–4
  hepatorenal syndrome 24
  varices 18–21
portal hypertensive gastropathy 21
portal vein thrombosis 18, 20–21
portal venous gas 3
portocaval shunts 20
portoenterostomy 48
portosystemic collateral circulation 18
portosystemic shunts 20, 23

praziquantel 32
prednisolone 15, 48
prerenal failure 24
primary biliary cirrhosis 1, 3, 17, 37
primary sclerosing cholangitis 3, 17
Pringle manoeuvre 28
proteolytic enzymes 33
prothrombin time 10
pruritis 17, 41, 43
pseudoaneurysms 40
pseudocysts, pancreatic 1, 34, 39–40
  pancreatic trauma 46
  ruptured 39

radiofrequency ablation 27
radiography 3
  acute pancreatitis 34
  chronic pancreatitis 38
  liver abscesses 29, 31
  pancreatic trauma 46
radiotherapy 43
Ranson's scoring system 34
renal failure
  acute pancreatitis 35
  hepatic encephalopathy 24
  pancreatic transplantation 47, 49
resuscitation 44
retinopathy, diabetic 49
retroperitoneal space
  bile staining 46
  necrosis 33
rheumatoid arthritis 15
rheumatoid factor 9
road traffic accidents 44, 46

schistosomiasis 18
scintigraphy 26
sclerotherapy 19
selenium 38
serum:ascites albumin gradient 22
shotgun injuries 44
sickle cell disease 1, 5
Sjögren's syndrome 17
sodium tetradecyl sulphate 19
sodium, dietary 22, 23
somatostatin 40, 43
somatostatin analogues 19
spherocytosis 1, 5
sphincter of Oddi division (sphincterotomy)
  8
  bile leaks 45
  gallstone pancreatitis 35, 36
spironolactone 23
splanchnicectomy, thoracoscopic 43
splenectomy 40
splenic artery pseudoaneurysms 40
splenic vein thrombosis 20–21, 40
splenomegaly 1, 9, 40
stab wounds 44
staphylococci 29
steatorrhoea 37, 38
stents 3
  acute cholangitis 6
  bile leaks 45
  common bile duct stones 8
  pancreatic carcinoma 42, 43

streptococci 29, 30

tacrolimus 48
terlipressin 19, 21
thalassaemia 1, 5
thrombocytopenia 25
thyroid disease 15
thyroid tumours 43
tilidine 38
total hepatic vascular isolation 45
tramadol 38
transjugular intrahepatic portosystemic shunt
  20, 21, 23
tribavirin 14
trientene 16
tubular necrosis, acute 24
tumour embolisation 27
tumour seeding 4, 26

ulcerative colitis 15, 17
ultrasound 3
  acute pancreatitis 34, 35
  ascites 22
  cholestatic non-obstructive jaundice
  16–17
  common bile duct stones 8
  cystic liver lesions 3, 25
  gall stones 3, 5, 6
  hepatocellular carcinoma 26
  hepatomegaly 3
  liver abscesses 29–30, 31
  liver biopsy 4
  pancreatic carcinoma 41
ursodeoxycholic acid 8, 17
urticaria 31

varices/variceal bleeding 18–21
  balloon tube tamponade 19–20
  band ligation 19
  cirrhosis 18
  endoscopy 19–20, 21
  gastric 21, 40
  hepatic encephalopathy 18, 20
  hepatitis B infection 13
  hepatocellular carcinoma 26
  liver transplantation 21
  oesophageal 18–21
  portal hypertension 18–21
  sclerotherapy 19
  splenic vein thrombosis 40
vasoactive peptide 43
vasopressin 19
vena cava lacerations 45
vitamin C 38
vitamin E 38
vitamin K 2
vitamin K_1 (phytomenadione) 18

Whipple's pancreaticoduodenectomy 39, 42,
  46
Wilson's disease 3, 15–16

xanthoma 17

zinc acetate 16